NATURAL

MEDICINE:

WHAT YOU NEED TO KNOW TO MAKE IT WORK FOR YOU

by

Pat O'Brien,
CAY, CCH, AADP, AHG

Disclaimer

The contents in this book are based on alternative methods and opinions derived from Ayurvedic and Chinese medicine, including the author's credentials and experience in practice. However, the information is in no way intended to be a substitute for the advice or diagnosis given to you by your licensed western medical doctor. The natural health information in this book is not meant to be a prescription. If you are on any prescription drugs or pregnant, consult a certified health-care practitioner before taking any herbs, as some could have consequences. All herbs and foods should first be researched thoroughly if you decide to use them. There is no 100% guarantee of a cure when using these methods. Futhermore, if you have a serious medical problem or life threatening emergency, you should consult a western physician or the nearest ER. By following the suggestions in this book, you are agreeing to do so at your own risk and personal responsibility. The author is not responsible for any consequences or adverse effects from following these suggestions.

ISBN 0-9742888-0-2 20.00

Library of Congress Control Number: 2003094201

Library of Congress Catalog Card Number:

Publisher: O'Brien, P.O. Box 264 Andover, NY 14806

author's website: www.realnaturalmedicine.com

I would like to thank Margaret Adams Rasmussen for all her help in coaching me in the steps necessary to get this book published. Hope Zaccagni did a great job in helping me design the book's front and back cover. Thank you, Hope! I would also like to thank Vicki Eaklor for her help editing this book, and for her support throughout the entire process.

This book is dedicated to all of the people in the world who are struggling to get physically well. My parents taught me some of life's most important lessons and philosophies including: never give up believing in your dreams, believing in yourself, and realize that almost anything is possible and attainable! My father was also the one who encouraged me to write this book. I am also grateful for all the wonderful experiences, sights, and sounds I have had, as well as the difficult roads I have taken and what they have taught me.

Contents

Introduction:

Why You Need This Book

This book is very special to me and I hope it will be as special to you. It contains answers to many of the questions people like you have concerning disease, health, and natural holistic methods. Since there is a huge number of publications available on the subject of natural medicine, many of you are probably confused as to what really works and what doesn't. Some fields of alternative medicine disagree with each other in their theories, leaving you with conflicting advice. However, there is no such thing as one "miracle cure" for all your ailments. Natural medicine is an extremely complicated field. Natural treatment that "really" works requires knowledge based on extensive years of study and research, and flexibility and an open mind to know when to break from the rules and theories rather than always relying on general information.

My Story

I studied specialized natural medicine for five years and have a private practice with 2 offices in New York State treating common medical disorders. I am a certified professional practitioner of Ayurvedic and Chinese natural medicine, board certified with the American Association of Drugless Practitioners, certified professionally with the American Herbalists Guild (which has serious requirements, including a peer review process), and a member of the Northeast Herbal Association. I am trained in Indian, Chinese and Western herbal medicine - a rare combination, as well as nutrition extensively! My certifications in Ayurveda come from the Bayville Ayurvedic Holistic Center on Long Island and the American Institute of Vedic Studies in Santa Fe, New Mexico. I studied traditional Chinese medicine and herbology through the Institute for Chinese Herbology in Oakland, California and the Connecticut Institute for Herbal Studies. At the Vega Institute in Oroville, California I studied with world-renowned guru Herman Aihara and was certified in macrobiotics. In 1998 and 1999, I was a featured writer for *Macrobiotics Today*, a magazine devoted to Chinese/macrobiotic medicine. In the earlier years of my life, I worked in the health supplement industry in three different states: Connecticut, Rhode Island, and New York. Today, in my practice, I am also referred to as a nutritionist, serious herbalist, and use countless vitamins, natural supplements, and natural home remedies such as salt baths, ginger compresses and pastes, etc., to heal the body and mind. Each year, I also lecture and give classes on various topics related to natural medicine and disease, particularly in the Northeast, as well as write magazine articles (see my website).

My pursuit of this profession is no surprise to me. I have always had a passion for natural medicine, nutrition, herbs, health, disease, athletics, and science since the ninth grade. Their relationship has always excited me. In fact, throughout junior high and high school, I was an athlete for tennis, swimming, basketball, track and cross-country. My passion for athletics and health led me to research the field of sports nutrition. This passion extended into my college years. While pursuing an undergraduate degree at Alfred University, I ran cross-country, and financed my education by working in the health food/supplement industry. I read almost everything on the market during that time, from concepts in Jethro Kloss's classic book: *Back to Eden*, to books on juicing, cleansing, raw food diets, enzyme therapy, vitamin therapy, and vegetarianism as well. In fact, I was a vegetarian for 13 years of my life! My first two years in college were spent as a biology/pre-med student before changing my major to philosophy. After college, I continued to run competitively in 5K races, while also employed as the Executive Director of the American Cancer Society. Following those years, I was employed in the mental health profession. Actually, when I reflect back on my earlier life, not a year went by in which I was either employed in the health profession in some way, or studying health as a student.

However, my serious study of natural medicine began in my early twenties when I became chronically ill. The Western medical profession's diagnosis was Epstein-Barr (Chronic Fatigue Syndrome). At that time, I also had recurring intestinal candida, and the common "oral thrush," along with irritable bowel syndrome, migraine headaches, the beginning of cartilage breakdown in my knees, severe insomnia, extreme exhaustion, low grade fevers, swollen lymph nodes, daily sore throats and was bleeding excessively between menstrual periods (sometimes two weeks at a time). What was most frustrating during this decade of my life was that I couldn't seem to recover. Young and chronically ill, I visited one medical doctor after another, all of whom were unable to help me because they couldn't determine what was exactly wrong. Standard medical tests on me always came back "normal." During a period of annoying urinary frequency, I even had x-rays because the traditional Western medical community had no idea what was causing my bladder to be so irritated and overactive. It was one of their diagnostic methods. In fact, they had approached my menstrual problems in the same manner. Several years later, I learned that in each case, the x-rays were totally unnecessary. I then tried one natural holistic practitioner after another, and watched my body develop new problems I never had. The nutritional and herbal recommendations I got repeatedly were poor, or too generalized for my body. Acupuncture treatments were no help to me either. I learned the hard way, during those years, that "natural" did not equal health. Just because something was natural, organic, or unprocessed, didn't mean it would help me, nor would standard recommendations for echinacea help boost my immune system, and ginseng prevent me from becoming run down without giving me headaches. General nutritional recommendations such as avoiding white sugar, sweet fruit juices and too much fruit in general, to combat yeast, didn't work for me. This advice made me temporarily hypoglycemic, which did show up on Western medical tests. In fact, within a year and a half of following this type of regime, I developed the beginning stages of jaundice, which concerned many. At one point, after following the advice of a holistic practitioner who was also an MD, I watched my hair fall out after taking certain herbs over a period of months. Since I was ignorant at the time, I had no idea that the herbal formulas and dietary recommendations that were given to me were the wrong ones. I trusted blindly the information I was given, never questioning anything. Nevertheless, it was only after I decided to pursue a profession as a natural health care practitioner, listen to my own advice and body, and take charge of my own health care, that I was able to recover.

Why General Advice Doesn't Work

Based on personal experience, being on every diet and natural supplement you can name while trying to achieve "health," and from my professional schooling and experience in private practice with patients, I will tell you up front that general advice doesn't work. It is too general! Simply to tell someone to take valerian for pain, or even garlic for high cholesterol is potentially dangerous, as the factors involved in a person's illness are complex and numerous. For example, because valerian is also a heating and pungent herb in its effects, not just a nerve sedative, it will exacerbate inflammatory types of pain, as heating substances aggravate inflammation in the human body's muscle and joint tissue. To recommend mega doses of vitamin C and orange juice for a cold when there is also a severe sore throat present, will feel like a death sentence - it would be like pouring gasoline on a fire. Vitamin C and orange juice are acidic (sour), and heating. A sore throat means localized inflammation and infection, and acidic and heating substances aggravate infection and inflammation. There are also dry type coughs with no mucus and more wet or damp types with heavy chest congestion and thick white mucus production. Many people assume all colds or "coughs" need to be cleared out, hence automatically take or prescribe decongestants and other substances to break up mucus. However, a dry cough will benefit from dairy products in the diet such as milk and ice cream, as well as plenty of fruit juices, as they are moistening to the human body and help lubricate dry mucous membrane tissues. But the latter type of cough with heavy congestion, will not. There are many generalizations, or beliefs about nutrition, herbs and natural supplements that are incorrect. In actual reality, people, their physical differences, illnesses, and the causes for those illnesses are much more complicated, hence the reason a natural therapy will often fail.

I will also tell you that to effectively treat disease naturally, considering all those complex variables, you need the information found in Ayurvedic and Chinese medicine. Due to many factors, I strongly believe that theses are the best natural medical systems in the world. Ayurvedic medicine alone, has a very deep and sophisticated level of understanding nutrition and herbology as a science beyond the well-known Western concepts of fats, proteins, carbohydrates, vitamins, and minerals. It also takes the energetic or chemical effects of a particular substance into account. Both Ayurvedic and Chinese medicine each have a very sophisticated and very effective way of looking at disease, diagnosing disease, and treating it. These medical systems gave me the answers to my own medical problems, and continue to help me treat my patients with an alarmingly high success rate. Ayurveda, in particular, has been the main alternative medical system responsible for my own recovery. Hence, the reason I chose to study it, and why it is the cornerstone of my practice and book. I am also biased towards Ayurveda as a superior natural medical system, because it even takes into account the genetic and physiological differences between people, hence predicting their disease tendency and dietary needs.

Additionally, both medical systems predate the Western U.S. medical system, and are also currently the most sought out and respected forms of natural medicine. Ayurveda is a 5000-year-old natural medical practice originating from India, and Chinese medicine is about 3000 years old. In India, Ayurvedic hospitals, pharmacies, and medical clinics still exist, offering alternative treatments for mild and serious medical conditions. In fact many physicians in India are considered MD's in Ayurvedic medicine. Ayurveda is also considered the mother of Chinese medicine, and several hospitals right now in the United States have Ayurvedic practitioners on staff including the 21st Century Hospital in Massachusetts and the New York University Alternative Medicine Facility for Health and Healing. As one in three people are now seeking holistic medicine as their primary form of treatment, more hospitals in the U.S. and world are moving towards integrative medicine, incorporating both natural medicine and Western medicine, including Ayurvedic medicine. The reason Chinese medicine is much more familiar to people in the United States is because it arrived here in this country first. It was the first natural medical system to get advertised.

Reversible Diseases and the Methods Used to Treat Them

Both systems, especially Ayurvedic medicine, have a very high success rate for treating and actually reversing disease. Contrary to what we have been taught, a lot of medical problems are indeed reversible. The fact that many people in America don't know this is due in part to Western medicine's view that some of those conditions are permanent, as the cause of those medical conditions are not yet understood. However, in Ayurvedic medicine, the cause for most medical disorders has been known for some time. Many disorders such as acid reflux, colitis, allergies, asthma and even inflammatory pain are reversible. Other treatable conditions, in many cases completely reversible, are: digestive system disorders such as irritable bowel syndrome, chronic constipation, ulcers, heartburn, intestinal candida/yeast, bloating and gas, nausea, diverticulitis; immune related disorders such as Epstein-Barr virus; food and environmental allergies, hay fever; some respiratory problems including recurring bronchitis, asthma; ear/nose/throat disorders especially chronic sore throats, sinusitis, and congested sinuses, ringing in the ears; reproductive disorders such as male impotence and premature ejaculation; female amenorrhea, menorrhagia (excessive bleeding), PMS, hot flashes, breast tenderness and swelling, dysmenorrhea/severe cramping, irregular menstrual cycles; heart disease/high cholesterol, hypertension/hypotension; hypoglycemia; hypothyroidism/hyper-thyroidism; nervous system disorders such as insomnia, depression, anxiety, and some types of tremors; weight loss/weight gain; poor circulation; anemia; skin disorders including acne, psoriasis, rosacea, and eczema; rheumatoid arthritis, gout, chronic urinary tract infections or any recurrent infections, some types of edema, fibromyalgia, and some types of back pain. In the case of osteoarthritis, I believe Ayurveda can halt the disease, not reverse it completely.

Furthermore, Ayurvedic and Chinese medicine treatment methods are gentle! Natural treatment is not invasive! It doesn't require being cut up, radiated or having to go through uncomfortable procedures in examination. The methods used to reverse or halt the disease process involve food/nutrition, herbal medicines, natural supplements, vitamins/minerals, lifestyle factors, exercise, counseling, color therapy, climate considerations, relationships, oil treatments, nasaya (herbs/medicated oils administered through the nasal passages), medicated herbal pastes called lepas, home remedies such as special baths and types of compresses, music, and aromatherapy. Treatment can incorporate anything for it involves everything and anything that can be an instrument in the healing and recovery process. In fact coffee can be used medicinally when used correctly in the right circumstances and case if appropriate. How so? Its properties are pungent, bitter, and heating. In certain cases of illness related to coldness or congestion and stagnation, it will increase circulation, warm the body, stimulate the nervous system, and help break up matter and mucus in the body. Did you know that chocolate is an anti-oxidant and contains magnesium? It is also a sweet, warming food that can help reduce muscle spasms. Also, black tea has just as many healing properties as green tea.

Anything can be an instrument in the healing process. Sugar can help cool hot flashes, and stop acidity in the gut, but when used either sparingly or excessively it can weaken the pancreas. What we put in our mouths and how we spend our day with certain types of activities, is a source of energy for us that can either help maintain our equilibrium or throw us off balance creating disease. The type of music we listen to, the type of relationships we have, and the TV movies we watch, all impact our health, especially our mental state. Nevertheless, all of the above can be a tool in the healing process or not.

While in some medical cases prescription drugs and surgery are valid choices for treating disease and may be necessary, they are not always the only or best choices to make. Sometimes alternative medicine can actually reverse the medical condition in a comfortable, natural, safer, as well as cheaper way. I have actually seen Ayurvedic medicine prevent surgery. However, it requires active participation on the patient's part, or change. This is what's called "active healing." The patient takes an active part in his/her own healing process, instead of a passive approach whereas they lie down, waiting for someone to "do it to them" and make them well. Once you have chosen this active approach, the results are very rewarding! You become extremely educated in the process, thus empowering yourself to be able to heal yourself the next time you need to.

However, because of the complexity of these fields, and the time required to learn it (which you may not have), I am giving you the most specific and vital information behind these two respected, ancient healing traditions so that you can try some of it yourself and get the answers that you need. I am saving you from having to read every book on the market in the field of holistic medicine, while making the same mistakes I once did. I have given you methods that have actually worked for real people who have sought my help as patients, and given you answers for why they worked, based on those experiences. *Natural Medicine: What You Need to Know to Make It Work For You* literally sorts the facts from the fiction. It shows you where most people make their biggest mistakes in natural health care. By becoming educated and learning how natural medicine really works, you will be able to get the best possible health care by making the best and most informed choices. You will regain power over your own health care, and be able to wisely choose natural supplements, herbs, and foods that really work for you. However, do realize that not seeing someone in person to be diagnosed professionally can limit somewhat the personalization of your own healing program and its accuracy that can be achieved, as one can misdiagnose themselves without enough information or schooling. For even more detailed and specific information on what therapies to use for your medical condition, seek a certified and knowledgeable health care practitioner for help, but always question those in authority! Check their backgrounds and schooling. Also, if something doesn't feel right, don't do it despite what someone else says! Trust yourself! Trust your body!

1

The Biggest Mistakes in Natural Medicine

What Natural Medicine is Really About

Natural medicine at its best teaches us about ourselves, our bodies, what we need or do not need. It empowers us to take control of our own health care and treat ourselves. It has a holistic approach that sees everything in the body as interconnected and related, including disease! The human body is also a microcosm, or a mini rendition of the macrocosm of the universe. From these perspectives, natural medicine sees illness simply as a state of imbalance in the body, mind, and spirit. Illness did not just come out of nowhere. We are no longer helpless victims who can do nothing in its face. Neither is illness some enemy to be fought and conquered. It teaches us where we went off course and how we have an opportunity to get back on, only this time going in another direction. We all fall out of balance or sync with ourselves from time to time. How much we fall out of balance is different for everybody and determines how ill we become. The greater the imbalance, the more severe the disease in the body. Health will then be restored when we restore our internal mental, spiritual and physical balance.

In fact, Indian and Chinese medicine share this view. Disease is basically a disharmony, and therefore eradicating the illness you have depends on treating the disharmony underlying the dysfunction of the organ, tissue, or system in your body. Therefore, it isn't necessary to name a disease or know what hormone is out of balance. If the disharmony pattern is recognized and treated, the dysfunction will go away and health will be restored.

What Optimal Health Looks Like

True health, from the holistic medicine perspective, includes not just "clean" medical tests, but dozens of visible signs harmony in the human body such as healthy digestion. This means no gas, nausea, or indigestion after eating; no abnormal hunger or lack of appetite; no undigested food particles in the feces; and neither diarrhea nor constipation. In Ayurveda, digestion is also a process by which many problems grow and branch out from. In addition, Ayurvedic medicine believes that harmony or "health" in the body is more likely to exist when the three main human wastes (urine, feces, and sweat) are also in a state of balance. This means that their production is neither deficient or excessive, as well as the fact that the urine should be normal colored like beer and the feces well-formed and floating.

Additional signs of health are: excellent, sound sleep not beyond eight hours per night, great physical stamina and energy, mental sanity free from true anxiety or depression, a good memory, a good temperament, no headaches, for women - a normal 5-day menstrual cycle that is 28-33 days apart with a moderate amount of blood and no severe cramps; no allergies, not catching frequent colds or the flu all the time, no nighttime urination or urinating frequently such as going to the bathroom 9-10 times a day, not feeling excessively cold or hot all the time, normal blood test results, no pain, no persistent symptoms of any kind, and no medically diagnosed disease/condition.

However, as most people in America already know, the definition of health from the Western medical perspective is quite different. I have often heard from my patients that their physicians told them they are in excellent health, yet they come to see me because they simply don't feel good. People have chronic headaches, chronic sinus infections, back pain, mouth canker sores, their menstrual period lasts three or 7-9 days, they have hot flashes, burning feet, muscle tension and pain, severe menstrual cramps, swollen fingers, insomnia, chronic depression, heart palpitations, bruise easily, premature hair loss, chronic diarrhea or loose stools, chronic bloating and gas in the abdomen, ringing in the ears, dizziness, itchy skin, rashes on their chest or arms, stomach pain right below the rib cage, nausea and frequent lack of appetite, etc. However, people with these symptoms often score "negative" results on Western medical tests. They have been through traditional medical tests such as x-rays, ultra sounds, blood tests, and upper and lower GI series tests. They have been scoped and pricked but nothing has been found to be biologically, chemically wrong with them; hence they are labeled "healthy." Yet they are uncomfortable or feel miserable, out of sync with themselves, and nobody seems to know what is wrong with them or what is causing their problems.

In holistic medicine, these symptoms are not signs of balance or health in the human body, they are the beginning symptoms of the disease process, hence they give practitioners clues as to what's wrong in an otherwise deemed "healthy" individual. One of the beauties of natural medicine is that it can spot trouble in the body that may not be perceivable on Western blood or traditional medical tests for some time until the disorder becomes severe.

Why Some People Don't Get Well Using Natural Methods

Ayurvedic and Chinese natural medicine make and use common sense in the treatment of disease. If a person has a problem that is caused from too much dryness in the body such as a dry flaky scalp (dandruff), or constipation, foods and herbal medicines that are moistening will help alleviate the problem. Excessive water retention in the tissues, such as certain types of edema, will lesson over time with herbs and foods that are drier or diuretic. Too much heat in the body, too much cold, tissue deficiency, blood deficiency, excessive mucus and congestion, will all benefit from herbs, foods, and natural substances that have energetic properties that are opposite in nature to that problem or that disperse that energy until the body returns to a state of balance, and hence health. If a person is too cold, make them warmer, too yin, make them more yang; if too heavy, make them lighter by adding in substances with more air and ether; if too acidic in the case of ulcers and heartburn, make them more alkaline, and vice versa. If they have loose stools caused from a damp condition (too much moisture in the body and watery foods in the diet), give them astringent substances that help bind and dry out the stools, and make their diet full of astringent, drier substances to prevent it from reoccurring. Foods, herbs, vitamins, minerals, lifestyle factors, climate temperature and humidity all have specific energetic and nutritional properties which in turn, affect the body and its chemistry in a certain way. These different chemical effects of nutritional substances are one main reason alternative medicine is so complicated.

Secondly, people are also biologically unique both mentally and physically. Some of us are heavier, some lighter. Some of us have tendencies towards dry skin, while others have thick skin as well as oily skin. Some people sweat more. We all think differently, gain and lose weight differently, walk differently, get sick differently, have different tones in our voices, and move at different speeds. When we have a bad day and are out of balance, some of us will lean towards anxiety, insomnia, or nervous energy, while some people will leans towards depression, and lethargy. Others will get irritated, ticked off and feel frustrated. Not all women who go through menopause will get hot flashes. Each female will experience menopause differently by having different symptoms based on her current state of balance or imbalance in her body at the time she enters menopause.

Third, because of these personal biological differences, each of us has different nutritional needs and higher requirements for certain foods, vitamins and minerals than others. Some of us have a greater biological need for calcium or vitamin C. This factor also explains why we all have different tastes for foods. We intuitively crave foods which help keep us in balance by fulfilling our unique nutritional requirements and needs for foods with certain properties. If we are in balance and in tune with our bodies, we will probably dislike drinking milk and eating oatmeal and winter squashes, if we are a naturally damp and somewhat heavier-built person (dairy products, oatmeal and winter squash are very damp, heavy foods). These concepts are the basis of Ayurveda. Knowing about yourself, your true nature, its tendencies, and characteristics, is invaluable information. When seeking out natural health care, one can make more effective choices with this type of information. This human "uniqueness" also explains why people don't recover after spending much effort, and helps them get the results they so much desire. Furthermore, knowing about your biological tendencies can help you predict how an herb or natural substance will affect you.

Last, most information does not account for or tell you that there are many different types of pain, different kinds of coughs, asthma, depression, arthritis, insomnia, etc. For example, as said earlier, a cough can be a dry hacking cough, one with thick white sputum/mucus, or one that has mucus that is blood streaked or tinted green and yellow. Depression can be due to too much internal dampness or heaviness in the tissues, a nerve chemical deficiency in the body, or environmentally related. Also, because of each person's biological differences, each person requires a specific treatment plan tailored to their unique body and medical condition to begin with.

The Six Most Important Secrets to Reversing Disease

Secret #1 Your Biological Uniqueness

The first key to demystifying illness is to recognize and to understand your biological (genetic) uniqueness. This concept is the fundamental belief of the Ayurvedic medical system. It can be your starting place. Once you've done this, you have taken the most important step in the journey of your recovery and are way ahead of the game. Your own health care is no longer a big mystery when you have a better understanding of how your body functions and is put together. The best natural medicine in the world is of little use if it is not right for your unique system. We are all physically different! You simply cannot take general advice, even if it is "natural," and expect to get well automatically if what you are putting into your body has the wrong substances in it for your body's unique system and medical condition.

I spent years eating natural unprocessed and some organic food. I also spent years eating so called "healthy" meatless alternatives such as tempeh, TVP, falafil, miso, and so on, but still could not get well. I took vitamins, minerals, digestive enzymes, acidophilus for yeast, ate brewers yeast, took cod liver oil, flaxseed capsules, mega doses of vitamin C, echinacea, ginseng, etc. I drank water with lemon squeezed into it. I tried ginger tea for nausea. I bounced from one health food store and holistic practitioner to the next, seeking information, trying one natural substance after another and still couldn't recover. I always took the wrong substances for my body, buying into the same advice on what's "healthy" that so many other people do. Even the information I was taught, earlier in my life, turned out to be incorrect. I read book after book and kept trying different programs and remedies. You simply cannot change the nature of your system or constitution. In Ayurvedic medicine this is referred to your body type or genetic makeup. We are all born with a unique genetic constitution that will be with us to the day we die. It largely predicts what diseases we are more susceptible to and explains why some of us dislike and cannot eat spicy foods, or digest beans, yogurt, broccoli, cauliflower, or cabbage without bloating and gas, etc. What changes over time, and on a day-to-day or month-to-month basis, is only our current state of balance or condition.

For example, if your body has a tendency to be acidic and sensitive to sour acidic substances (you dislike their taste and digest them poorly - they give you gas or bloating), then natural vitamins, supplements, herbs and even foods that are acidic/sour will never help you! Apple cider vinegar, yogurt, grapefruit, strawberries, umeboshi plums, and vitamin C (which fall into this category) will never be health foods for you. It's a law of nature. If you have excessive yeast in your intestinal tract or constant oral thrush, and happen to be an acidic body type, then acidophilus tablets, miso, and tempeh will never help you combat yeast! These are all fermented substances and fermented foods are considered sour or acidic in Ayurveda. Sour substances tend to ferment in the digestive tracts of certain individuals, who are not designed to digest them! It is this excessive fermentation that causes yeast! If you ignore this fact of nature, your body will continue to remain out of balance, and you may develop chronic health problems.

Every single person on this planet has certain physical limitations, and when they violate them, they risk getting sick! If you have a biological tendency to be thin and have dry skin and hair, then foods, herbs, and substances that are drying in their properties, won't help you. They can't possibly be health foods for you, especially if you have a medical problem related to too much dryness in your system such as dry coughing or wheezing. Dairy products, melons, and bananas, will not help an individual who has a biological tendency to retain water very easily, gain weight easily, or often produce heavy, damp mucus during colds; nor will tofu be a health food for the person with a cold, damp, mucusy type of asthma. If strong hot spices give you diarrhea every time you eat them, then plain straight ginger tea, as a natural treatment remedy for nausea, may be too strong for you! Ginger is hot! Therefore, it is of utmost importance that you grasp this concept: "Healthy" is a relative term.

One person's medicine may also be another's poison. As stated above, we are all different and unique. We have different genetics, different mind types/personalities, different digestive tracts, different nutritional needs, different exercise requirements, different lifestyles and different herbal needs too. We all process stress differently. Hence seven different people with the same illness should receive different treatments and recommendations. Therefore, healing naturally should always be personalized to be the most effective. This is why thousands of people take vitamin C for the common cold or an infection, but only some experience benefits from taking it. For some people, it aggravates their system, especially if they already have an ulcer, colitis, heartburn, or strep throat (all which can be aggravated by acidic substances). Vitamin C is acidic in its properties, hence its sour taste. Sour substances can feed acidic and inflammatory conditions, including vinegar and lemon juice squeezed in water. However, in other people, vitamin C is the very substance they need.

Another example is the herb echinacea. This herb has been used among many people to boost the immune system at the onset of a cold or flu. It has excellent antibiotic (infectious fighting) properties. However, in some individuals, this herb can cause dizziness, insomnia, feeling “hyped up," and feeling depleted in terms of energy, if used in large enough dosages and for extended periods of time. This is due to the fact that the herb is a bitter, and bitter substances are catabolic (break down tissue and the body’s system eventually). Bitters fight infection, but do not “build up” the body and can actually weaken the immune system over a long period of time, especially in an individual who is already frail, weak, and tends towards deficiency related health problems. The key to strengthening the immune system is not the same for everyone! Everybody's system works differently and is strengthened in different ways. This is also the reason why scientifically testing herbal medicine on people in clinical trials is so difficult. If you take the wrong herbs, the wrong natural supplements, and eat the wrong foods for your unique body chemistry and medical condition, you can not get well. It's almost that simple and a fact, and the main reason people do not succeed at treating their illness naturally.

Secret #2 Treating the Root Cause

The second tool that I am going to share with you is that in order to reverse disease, you must treat its root cause. Without doing this, you cannot expect to recover. The disease symptoms will only be masked, so that you temporarily don't feel their discomfort. This is why people try different forms of natural medicine and don't get better or keep coming back for more treatments and appointments. By ignoring the root cause of an illness, the problem is likely to keep reappearing or travel to a different area of the body. When it does this, it pops out somewhere else. For example, if an infectious inflammatory condition caused chronically infected tonsils and the tonsils were surgically removed without addressing the cause, the infection/inflammation is likely to travel in the body to other tissues and appear as high fevers, inflammatory pain, or skin rashes, etc., depending on a variety of circumstances.

Simply treating the symptoms has been the American approach to health care for a long time. This approach is something we are accustomed to, and for some people it interferes with their ability to try alternative medicine. People are used to quick results that "hide" the true problem, and then give up if they don't experience immediate relief. Treating illness at the root requires time. For example, coffee is used in our society sometimes for fatigue besides taste. It perks the person up because of its caffeine content affecting blood sugar and metabolism. A person who drinks coffee all day long will not really feel the fatigue unless they stop the coffee because the coffee is "masking" the fatigue. So while it seems like an immediate solution, coffee does not treat the root cause of the problem. Had that individual been on a treatment program, several months later the fatigue may have completely banished or decreased!

Americans are geared towards expecting immediate solutions and instant gratification. When a man or woman has a headache, they take an aspirin and the pain is gone in an hour or so. When a woman has two weeks of nonstop menstrual bleeding, but no sign of cancer, tumors, fibroids, or anything unusual, she is given hormone pills, a D&C, or in some rare cases a hysterectomy. When she starts the hormone pills, the bleeding stops almost immediately. However, the underlying problem is still there and resumes when she stops the medication, just like the person who continues to get headaches on a weekly basis and continually pops aspirin or other pain relievers. The headache never truly disappears.

However, while natural medicine may sometimes be the better choice, treating the root cause is much slower. This is often why people give up. They give up too soon and expect miracles. The time involved to reverse a medical condition depends on many factors from the depth it has reached in the body, the actual tissue layer, organ or area of the body involved, to the level of participation on the patient's part and number of months or years they've had the illness. Some illnesses are also more complicated than others and involve more than one causal factor or pattern of disharmony. Recovery using natural methods can take one to seven or eight months depending on the case. However, when the problem does leave naturally, it is likely to stay away for some time, and the rewards are very gratifying if you hold out!

Secret #3 More Than One Cause for the Same Medical Condition

The third secret I want to share with you, is that there is more than one cause for what appears to be the same medical condition. For example, anemic conditions of the body can be brought on by what Chinese and Ayurvedic natural medicine call deficiency in the body (deficient blood in Chinese medicine), or from uterine hemorrhaging or heavy menstrual bleeding during the period. Weak veins and vessels leaking blood can also bring on anemia. Therefore, the treatment approach should be different in each case to bring about the most effective healing. Simple giving the person iron tablets, in the second case above, is not going to bring about a permanent cure unless the person addresses what is causing the heavy bleeding to begin with, and works at stopping the bleeding. Insomnia, arthritis, asthma, allergies, and fatigue have several different causes as well, since there are several different types of each. To effectively reverse a medical problem, you must know the specific type you have. For example, you must learn to differentiate between the subtle variations and types of a cough/cold. There are dry types of coughs, coughs with infection present, and damp types with much mucus and sputum. Not all types need to be "cleared out" of the head. In many cases people make the mistake of immediately removing dairy from the diet, assuming the cough is a damp one. Dry types actually benefit from milk, ice cream, and sweet juices - all of which help restore moisture back into the body.

Secret #4 Choosing the Wrong Supplements

The fourth secret is that most people use the wrong products, whether it's herbal formulas, natural supplements, vitamins, or foods. They do this because they take the label information on the product literally and all inclusively. Since, it's impossible to fit a lot of information on a tiny label, most companies will do their best by listing a general recommendation for that product. The fact that there is more than one cause and variation for most medical conditions means that you simply can't pick a product solely based on the label.

A good example of this is the many digestive aids on the market. The majority of these supplements have labels on them indicating that they are for the treatment of digestive complaints or "poor digestion." However, poor digestion can mean a variety of different things such as: chronic heartburn, diarrhea, constipation, bloating/gas, or nausea. Each one of these conditions requires a different treatment approach and of course different herbs, supplements, and dietary advice. For example, betaine hydrochloric acid and digestive enzyme tablets increase acid and enzyme secretions in the gut, which is bad news if you have heartburn, or an ulcer. When you increase these types of secretions in the stomach, you not only change your pH, but also increase the rate in which food material moves through your intestinal tract, making disorders like diarrhea and colitis worse. General recommendations for chamomile or peppermint for all digestive complaints, are not always helpful either, as these herbs can aggravate or cause bloating and gas in some people. What causes one person to develop bloating and gas in their intestinal tract verses another will be completely different. In some people, spicy, fermented, and sour foods cause it. In others, dry foods like beans, broccoli, and popcorn cause it.

Secret #5 Diseases Are Often Related

The fifth secret I want to share with you is that because the upper and lower body and human mind are related and interconnected as one whole unit, illnesses are often related. In Ayurveda (Indian) and Chinese medicine, diseases usually fall on specific patterns of disharmony. The same disharmony that caused a person to develop one medical problem, may be causing the other problems he/she has. For example, in Ayurveda hot flashes fall along the same pattern as high fevers, burning types or inflammatory arthritic pain, some types of skin rashes, and sometimes, but not always, certain kinds of diarrhea and tonsillitis. They are a disorder related to an imbalance of the biological humor pitta in the system. In Chinese medicine they are seen as part of a heat pattern.

Another example, in Ayurveda, involves a vata disharmony, in which there is a deficiency of the lack of fluids, blood, or plasma in the body. This type of dryness in the body can also cause dry lips, dry mouth, dry skin and eyes, cause the hair to fall out, the spine to crack as the synovial fluid dries up, chronic constipation, and the urine volume to diminish.

A third example is a pattern in which dampness pervades the tissues and systems in the body due to high kapha. It may first become evident as simply extra weight gain, a sweet sticky taste in the mouth, thick saliva, loose stools, and heavy sweating. Then what may develop or become more noticeable is a damp type of asthma or difficulty breathing in humid weather, a heavy feeling in the limbs, damp type arthritis, and finally edema (swelling) in the legs, around the knees, breasts and ankles.

In Chinese medicine, a liver disharmony, can cause these types of symptoms in an individual: chronic headaches, breast soreness right before the onset of the menstrual period, anger, irritability, frustration, an irregular menstrual cycle, genetic high cholesterol, neck and shoulder muscle tension, and pain or tenderness over the liver area below the rib cage.

Secret #6 Small Problems Can Turn Into Serious Health Problems

The sixth secret is that health problems that started out as small minor inconveniences can also turn into bigger illnesses as a result of being part of the same disease pattern. Basically, a minor symptom, that has progressed when left unchecked and allowed to flourish in the body for some time, can then become a much more severe medical problem. The chances of an illness progressing can be high, especially if the person continues the same dietary and lifestyle habits that caused the problem to occur in the first place. For example, a condition that started out as chronic constipation, dry mouth, lips and sinuses, chronic fatigue, low body weight, hyperactivity and insomnia (excessive dryness in the body, along with tissue deficiency and wind in the nervous system - a vata disorder in Ayurveda), and ignored for a long time, might turn into cracking in the joints, hair loss, deficient menstrual blood, more severe insomnia, and/or tremors in the hands. As dryness augments in the body, it wrecks havoc by drying up the body's vital fluids including menstrual blood and synovial fluid in the joints. When it is localized in the respiratory passages, it can create some types of allergies, particularly to dust and smoke, and even "dry asthma." Severe tissue deficiency combined with chronic dryness in that individual, could also set that person up for ammenorrhea (cessation of the menstrual period) or osteoarthritis (a condition in which cartilage breaks down in the joints).

In a different example, a simple case of feeling cold all the time with cold hands and feet, can turn into a mysterious condition of urinary frequency (abundant clear and copious urine) because the body will excrete more urine more often as a way to warm up. Other symptoms that may go along with a cold imbalance in the system are: a pale complexion and tongue, a slow pulse, nighttime urination, possible diarrhea, edema, and even lower back pain, as muscles sometimes contract from internal cold in the body. In Chinese medicine, we would say a pattern of kidney yang deficiency (coldness and weakness in the kidney and bladder area), is developing.

In a third example, a person with chronic acid indigestion and hot flashes can more easily develop an ulcer, be more susceptible to frequent infections such as sinus infections, develop chronic sore throats, and even inflammatory pain, as increased acidity and heat in the body combine to help create this disease pattern. However, by simply being aware of these patterns, and many others, you can use this invaluable information to help you get clues to determine the cause of your illness or problem!

What Practitioners Secretly Want to Know About You

So how do Ayurvedic and Chinese practitioners determine the root cause and disease patterns in your body, or your biological uniqueness? They rely on many different clues to help make an accurate diagnosis of your medical condition. Since holistic medicine does not rely on traditional Western methods to make a diagnosis, most people always ask me what methods are used instead. In an hour or two session, a holistic practitioner asks extensive questions to get a picture of your current life, your background, and medical history, take the pulses to determine the underlying imbalance, and do a physical examination of the hair, hands, gums, tongue, face, skin, abdomen, etc.

When feeling your pulse, a practitioner of Ayurvedic or Chinese medicine will feel its speed (is it fast or slow), look at its strength (is it pulsating strong like a frog under the fingers or is its pressure weak, thready); check its tempo (moving rhythmically slow and gracefully like a swan; or irregular, fast, or choppy). Is your pulse felt only at the superficial level (top layer right under the fingers), or can it be felt strong at the deep third level when more pressure is applied? Is your pulse thick or thin, wiry, slippery, etc.? Under each finger, a practitioner may even look for the imbalance within a particular organ, as the organs have their respectable pulse positions. Hence, the reason you always see an Ayurvedic or Chinese practitioner apply three fingers to your wrist. For example, on the left wrist, the second position denotes gall bladder and liver function.

As your tongue is examined, the practitioner looks at its coloration; whether there is any coating on the tongue; the location, thin or thickness, and color of the coating; whether your tongue has any cracks on it, is it peeled and dry, swollen, scalloped on the edges, or is there a tremor in it. Your hair will be examined to see if it is dry, brittle, if you have split ends, whether it is shiny, oily, or falling out, and whether your scalp is flaky, dry, or red. Your face will be examined for color, whether it is gaunt, pasty, swollen, red, has acne, rosacea or dry scabies on it, and how you wrinkle.

Then the practitioner will pay attention to your gate, the sound of your voice, your physical movements, ask about your physical stamina, your activity level, and try to form a mental picture of your lifestyle. Furthermore, they may ask about the nature and color of your stools, color and frequency of your urine, the taste in your mouth or thickness of your saliva, the type of mood swings you have, and the characteristics of the cough you have (Is it a dry cough you have or a one with mucus? What color is the mucus and is it thick or thin?). They want to know if your sleep is heavy or interrupted. Do you have trouble going to sleep? They also want to know about your occupation, relationships and home environment to help determine whether your problems are purely physical or environmentally related. They also care about the nuisances you have, such as headaches, backaches and the specific type of pain you experience. Is it a dull aching pain, a burning pain, or sharp stabbing pain?

These kinds of questions and observations are necessary for a proper diagnosis. The answers to these questions, as well as the nature of your pulse, tongue, skin, etc., help determine the possible disharmonies in the body and their patterns. The most detailed and accurate picture of you can be gotten from seeing you in person. A practitioner can palpate certain areas of your body to feel for heat, cold, texture, swelling, and look at the coloration and location of the problem. Your abdomen, torso, and other regions might be palpated to check for any tenderness. However, what follows in the next section, are tools to help you put the best possible picture together of yourself, without seeing someone in person. Determining your "biological blueprint" is one of the most important pieces of information you can have to help solve the riddle of your illness and prevent it from coming back.

2

Your Biological Blueprint and Disease Tendency

What is a Biological Blueprint?

In order to really help you begin to help yourself, it is first necessary to go into some information about Ayurveda and the physical and mental differences between people. These differences make up your biological blueprint (genetics)- basically the things that make you "tick." In Ayurveda there are different categories of specific physical and mental characteristic traits that people usually fall into, making people different among each other. Each category is governed by a "dosha." There are three doshas called "vata," "pitta," and "kapha." The doshas are irreducible invisible forces that govern the physical and mental body giving people their specific characteristics, and they can even cause disease. Generally speaking, vata dosha governs all movement in the body, things like nerve impulses, and involuntary breathing; pitta is responsible for things like body temperature, the skin, the blood, liver activity, the endocrine system, digestion/ metabolism; and kapha is involved in building and maintaining the structures of our bodies. It helps create plasma, synovial fluid in the joints, connective tissue, bone and so on. These three forces or "doshas" help make up the human body by being responsible as the catalysts in all the cellular activity that occurs. In addition to that, each dosha within us, also has its own unique set of specific characteristic traits that affect activity in the body in some way, including the state of our health.

Vata is the category or force in the body that has certain qualities such as coldness, dryness, roughness, and sharpness. It is responsible for making the body more alkaline, creates movement, is responsible for speed, is subtle, can be irregular, clear, and creates lightness in the body such as low weight and airiness. It is considered the "wind" or hollowness of the body. It is the space in the body's channels, and is what makes nerve impulses happen. As stated above, vata dosha is responsible for all cellular movement in the body, and mechanical actions including the automatic response of breathing in and out.

Pitta is and has the characteristic of being acidic, sour, sharp, hot, moist, oily, and light. It helps keep the body warm, controls temperature, and is considered part of blood and the waste product of blood. It is the

acid that digests our food. When pitta is too high in the body, a person's system is usually too acidic or over heated. Pitta is also bile, hence its seat in the liver as well. Since this dosha governs metabolism and helps create appetite, it is closely associated with "fire."

Kapha has the qualities of always being damp, cold, sticky, static, sweet, heavy, slimy, slow, oily, stable, soft, and dull. These attributes help the body build matter and material such as bone, and cartilage. Kapha also gives the body its fat and cushions the joints with its wet, sticky, soft material. Phlegm is a kapha material, hence kapha's association with water. Kapha's moisture is needed in the body to create blood and plasma.

We all have all three doshas (vata, pitta, kapha) inside of us, as these are necessary for human life. However, some of us tend to have one dosha or two in greater quantity than others that predominates and hence has a tendency to be in excess. Your unique body type is based on which dosha that tends to dominate giving you your biological uniqueness. When there is more of one dosha in greater quantity than the others in the body, that person is likely to have more physical characteristics of that dosha. For example, if you are a kapha predominate individual, you will have a genetic tendency to gain weight easily, retain water, or medical "edema," due to kapha's heavy, moist, and anabolic qualities. If you get sick, you are more likely to get chest colds, or coughs with heavy thick mucus. Pitta people will tend be medium weight, are more sensitive to heat, and develop more easily disorders related to acidity such as acid flux disease, due to the heating and acidic qualities of pitta. Vata predominate people will have a tendency to be underweight, as well as having dry physical characteristics, such as dry skin and hair, and tendencies towards chronic constipation (dryness in the colon), and so on. These tendencies are due to vata's dry nature.

However, most people are "mixed" types, or a combination of two dominating doshas. If you have two doshas in near equal quantity, then you are a "dual doshic" person or mixed body type. In my opinion, there are about nine different dosha combinations (body types) that people will usually fall into. Their names are: vata, vata-kaphavata-pitta, pitta-vata, pitta, pitta-kapha, kapha-pitta, kapha, and tridoshic (having equal parts of vata-pitta-kapha). A vata-pitta individual will have slightly more vata physical and disease tendencies, and secondarily pitta ones, whereas in a pitta-vata person, pitta will dominate, but vata will also be part of their makeup to a lesser extent. However, remember that no two people are exactly alike. So even two people of the same dual doshic body type, like vata-pitta, can be somewhat different in their physical makeup. One may be a cold, acidic type, and the other may be a warm and more alkaline type.

How and Why You Get Sick

These three forces (doshas) must remain in balance to create health. How and why you develop the illnesses you do, depends a lot on your diet, lifestyle, environment factors, the uniqueness of your body/genetic type as mentioned above, and whether your doshas are in a state of balance. Ever wonder why some people always get chest colds or colds with a lot of congestion, some seem to get sore throats all the time and others always get a dry hacking cough, or suffer from insomnia? In Ayurveda, the body type you have (or "doshic" combination), largely predisposes you to certain diseases/imbalances. This factor explains why one person gets heartburn more easily because of their higher acid production and so on. Some argue that genetics play a role in everything including disease. This is true because people in families tend to pass on their genetic coding to their children/offspring and hence the children tend to have similar body types as the parents. What is also true, is that people in families or from the same families tend to have similar eating and living habits, as well as similar attitudes about life. However, people tend to have doshic imbalances that are related to their genetic type, as this is the strongest and hardest factor to control, although this is not always the case each time.

For example, kapha people have a genetic tendency to get kapha related diseases, and vata/pitta people tend to develop vata/pitta related health problems. However, a vata predominate person can also develop pitta related heath problems such as an ulcer or migraine. And a kapha person can have a pitta type of arthritis such as inflammatory type pain. What is also true is that people who have a tendency to eat things that aggravate their body type or doshic imbalance (medical condition), stay sick. For example, if you are a kapha, when sick, your kapha might be in excess. This means that if you have a natural tendency to be internally cold and damp, a kapha health problem for you may mean your innate dampness, cold, and heavyqualities are in excess, possibly causing a damp type of asthma, allergies, or excess congestion, in the form of a chest cold, in your body. Your body might be producing an abundance of mucus, some water retention or excess weight because of its damp, heavy, oily, and sticky attributes. The high kapha in the system may even be the extra water that is causing a woman's breast tissues to swell right before her menstrual period, or why the tissues surrounding her ankles tend to pool water. To be in a state of balance, if you are a kapha predominate person, then means to keep your dampness in control and within a normal level. One way to do that is by avoiding damp foods, damp herbs, and heavy substances.

Another example of how these principles work is: if vata's qualities of lightness or speed are increased, then a person who already has these biological tendencies may experience unwanted weight loss (fast metabolism and wasting of the body's tissues), a fast resting heart rate, hyperactivity or restlessness, heart palpitations, and even some types of tremors. Excess lightness and windy qualities of vata in the body, can also cause ringing in the ears (as one cause of ringing in the ears, in Ayurveda, is from trapped air and ether in the ear and nerve channels). If the inherently dry qualities of vata were to increase, then a person might start to see the skin, mouth, or sinuses becoming dry, maybe a diminished flow in urine volume, dandruff (dry scalp), cracking in the joints and spine, as fluids dry up in these areas, hard stools or constipation, and possibly a scanty menstrual flow (light period) if the person is female.

With pitta in excess in the body, extra heat and/or acidity can cause hot flashes, frequent infections or high fevers, ulcers, bleeding disorders such as excessive and prolonged menstrual bleeding, or gingivitis. The appetite might also be increased since an increase in digestive enzyme activity and heat, "digestive fire," would be prevalent. Heat in the body also drives up thirst as heat burns up fluids, so an increase in pitta in the body can cause a person to have excessive, abnormal thirst. Remember, health is a state of balance; the absence of symptoms and the balance of the three doshas.

Determining Your Biological Blueprint and Disease Tendency

To help you determine your biological blueprint (doshic makeup), there is a short list following of some of the physical and mental characteristics associated with the doshas. Check off what best describes you from each doshic category, pick the category (ies) in which you scored the most, and then use that information as one guideline to knowing something about your own body type. If you checked off mostly vata traits, then it is likely that you have a lot of vata in your system by birth or a vata imbalance at the moment. If you checked off equal amounts of vata and pitta traits, then you may be dual doshic and a vata-pitta. If you checked off slightly more pitta than vata traits, but vata runs a close second, you may be a pitta-vata type person. If this was reversed, you would most likely be a vata-pitta person, having slightly more vata traits than pitta.

Also read what follows after the doshic test, and note the physical diseases tendencies that each of the three main category/doshic types are likely to get when unbalanced. Circle the medical problems you have had, in each of the categories. How you get sick over and over again has a lot to do with which dosha is constantly imbalanced. This is another big clue or indicator of your body/genetic type, as most people tend to get medical problems related to their body makeup, as I stated before.

Use this information also as a guideline when making food selections for yourself. Choose foods that can help keep your dosha(s)/natural biological tendencies in balance. In part 6, also look up the health problem you have and use the information about your body type and current doshic symptoms (imbalance), when selecting natural treatment methods, including herbs. Remember, the same herb or supplement should not be used for everyone just because they have the same medical problem from observation. People are different and there are different manifestations of the same illness. For example, there are actually three main kinds of arthritis (vata, pitta, kapha) and many more minor variations such as pitta-kapha, or pitta-vata arthritic symptoms. If you do not have a clear understanding about your own nature (prakruiti or body type), make an appointment with a certified and reputable Ayurvedic practitioner.

Checklist to Help You Determine Your Body Makeup

Your sleep has a tendency to be:

Vata – very light, interrupted, about 6-7 hours, sometimes you have insomnia and can't fall back to sleep or have trouble getting to sleep
Pitta – moderate, 7-8 hours
Kapha – heavy, 8-10 hours, sometimes you nap during the day or you have trouble waking up in the morning because you feel lethargic and groggy, it takes you several hours after waking up to feel mentally alert, or you need coffee to wake up.

Your body shape:

Vata – slim, trouble gaining weight, tubular shaped, almost like Ken and Barbie with no hips/narrow hips and a flat or small chest
Pitta – medium build, you can gain and lose weight with effort, chest and hip size are medium, you are athletic or muscular looking
Kapha – women have Goddess/voluptuous/pear shapes, thick arms and thighs, large breasts, gain weight easily and have a hard time losing it; men have broad shoulders, thick arms and legs, a hard time losing weight; always seem to carry a lot of fat and were chubby or stocky throughout most of life

Your thighs and arms have a tendency to be:

vata – thin, spindly, have underdeveloped muscles
pitta- medium sized, muscular
kapha– thick, heavy, can't see the muscles underneath

Your bowel movements/digestion:

Vata – tendency towards constipation; broccoli and granola give you bloating and gas
Pitta – loose oily stools or diarrhea, sometimes gas; sour and fermented foods bloat you up
Kapha – thick, soft, bulky stools that move out slowly, can digest and eat almost anything

Your appetite:

Vata – irregular, sometimes hungry, sometimes not
Pitta – always hungry, huge appetite, love to snack and eat at night or anytime, hate to miss a meal, occasionally experience sour burping or a sour taste in the mouth
Kapha – can fast for long periods of time and feel physically great, appetite variable also, sometimes feel nauseous, or have a sticky sweet taste in the mouth or thick saliva

Your moods when out of balance:

Vata - tendency towards anxiety, hyperactivity, easily excited, nervous, fearful, impulsive
Pitta - get irritated, frustrated and angry easily, you want to "get even" with the world

Kapha - laid back, happy or depressed, lethargic, want to hibernate or isolate, easy going

When sick with a cold, flu or virus, you usually develop:

Vata – dry scratchy throat, dry hacking coughs, laryngitis, watery and clear dripping mucus, dull, achy pain that changes its location often
Pitta – sore throats, strep throat, fevers, coughs with green, yellow, or blood-streaked mucus, burning or inflammatory type pain, you also get infections easily like sinus infections or bronchitis
Kapha – chest colds, heavy, thick, white mucus, abundant phlegm, heavy dull aching pain

Climate that bothers you the most:

Vata – cold, windy, or dry weather such as the fall season, or desert climate of Arizona
Pitta – hot, humid weather like the climate of Florida
Kapha – cold, damp/wet weather like spring, winter and rainy seasons

Skin texture and temperature:

Vata – thin skin, dry, flaky, cracked, rough, prominent veins, cold hands and feet
Pitta – sunburn easily, fair skin or skin with red blush, slightly oily, stay warm easily, sometimes feel too hot, hate the summer heat

Kapha – thick, moist skin, pale/pasty, oily, cold skin, sweat easily in large amounts

Your hair texture seems to be:

Vata – dry or sparse
Pitta – fine
Kapha – thick and oily, needs washing frequently

Your voice:

Vata - high pitched or soft
Pitta – argumentative, or strong, you speak with authority or strong opinion
Kapha – deep voice, but you speak rather pleasantly

You prefer the taste of these types of foods:

Vata: sweet, sour, and salty foods such as oatmeal, pancakes, sweet potatoes, coconut, bananas, lemons, kiwis, tomatoes, granny smith apples, yogurt, sour cream, pickles, vinegar, fish

Pitta: sweet, astringent, and bitter foods such as red apples, pears, cherries, grapes, oatmeal, winter squashes, white potatoes, broccoli, cauliflower, chickpeas, kidney beans, lettuce, spinach

Kapha: pungent, bitter, astringent foods like radishes, onions, leeks, eggplant, most legumes, white potatoes, broccoli, carrots, apples, pears, peaches, berries, salads, peas, collard greens, rye bread, cornbread, strong spicy spices

Personal habits/likes/dislikes:

Vata – you dislike routine, feel restless and have to be moving/doing something, are physically active, eccentric, like art, music, plays, you are a risk taker
Pitta – love to play sports, are athletic, driven, competitive, like the outdoors, camping, prefer cool fresh air, are a leader type, women may be tomboys
Kapha – you would rather read a book, watch TV, relax, sleep until noon, spend a night at a luxurious hotel and have breakfast in bed, you prefer solitude and quiet

Your scores:

vata ____________

pitta ____________

kapha ____________

Your Disease Tendency

As seen above, each dosha has its own set of characteristics and because of that, disease will manifest differently depending on the dosha that's involved, as well as causing people to have certain biological or genetic differences in their physical makeup, and different mental personalities.

For example, since vata has characteristics of being fast, dry, rough, cold, unstable/changing, moving, and lightness in the body, vata predominant people often feel hyperactive or restless and fidgety, like to be on the go. They tend to be eccentric, artsy, imaginative people who are generally thin most of their entire lives. They tend to suffer from tissue deficiency more easily than other types of people, hence they have trouble gaining weight when they want to. Their body tends toward catabolism. Their cheeks can become sunken in extreme cases, as the fat leaves their bodies. They have minds that never stop thinking, worry a lot, are small or flat-chested, burn out easily since their stamina is often poor, and tend towards anxiety, insomnia, and heart palpitations.

When sick, they have a tendency towards diseases related to deficiency in the body and internal dryness such as: dry hacking coughs, laryngitis, dandruff, hair loss, and dry cracked skin, dry lips, dry sinuses, a dry or cracked tongue, dehydration, and constipation. Therefore, the vata person is most sensitive to dry climates such as that of the fall seasons or desert regions. The women tend to have light scanty menstrual periods and deficiency types of anemia. Men are prone to impotence due to qi ("chi") deficiency, lack of strength and stamina. Diseases and imbalances due to wind (too much air and ether) in Chinese medicine are most common in vatas. Lockjaw, ringing in the ears, some types of tremors, spasms, some types of dizziness and Parkinson's disease are vata wind related illnesses. Vata people are also more likely to develop diseases due to deficient qi (lack of vitality), collapsed qi such as prolapsed organs, deficient plasma, deficient blood, and general coldness. Some other vata disorders are leg cramps, colic/gas (abdominal bloating), and some but not all types of anemia. Osteoarthritis is a vata disorder.

Vata type people leans towards being more alkaline and hence need a more acidic diet (such as eating plenty of tomatoes, lemons, and taking vitamin C) to keep their immune systems in balance. They should avoid foods which promote a catabolic nature in the body or substances which are simply too drying such as: broccoli, cauliflower, cabbage, kale, peas, too many salads, beans/legumes, cornmeal, corn chips, rye bread, buckwheat, and tea as a beverage.

Pitta people are the athletes in society and look good in preppy clothes because of their medium, muscular or square shaped bodies. They often get agitated, irritated and angry easily, like to argue or fight, and are short tempered. They often walk with determination. Because of their fair skin, they sunburn easily. Their physical weakness lies in the fact that they are susceptible to heat and acid conditions such as: inflammation, infections, blood related health problems, sore throats, strep throat, diarrhea/loose stools, canker sores, ulcers, skin disorders such as acne, rosacea, eczema, psoriasis; bleeding heavily during the menstrual cycle, and spotting or bleeding between menstrual periods. Colitis, heartburn, jaundice, and hepatitis are pitta related illnesses. Blood in the urine or sputum sometimes indicates infection, or heat, hence high pitta. Because of this tendency to have inflammatory/fire, and/or acid type problems, pitta people often experience "burning" or strong throbbing pain when they get arthritis. Hot flashes, fevers, and a voracious appetite and thirst, are common. Pitta people often suffer from what the Chinese call “yang”-related illnesses. In true pitta heat patterns, the tongue and face will become somewhat red and the pulse will be more rapid. Hot humid weather is the most aggravating to the pitta person.

Stagnant liver qi disharmonies (when the energy of the liver doesn’t flow properly) are common in pitta people causing disorders such as irregular menses to genetic high cholesterol. Sour burping, sour taste in the mouth, are all pitta traits and signs of an imbalanced liver as well. Other liver related problems include migraines, frequent headaches, or having sore breast tissue right before or during the menses.

Also importantly, these people simply cannot digest fermented foods, sour foods, or tolerate hot spices without developing bloating, gas and diarrhea from consuming them. Hence they should minimize them, along with avoiding too much vitamin C. Fermented substances, including yogurt, acidophilus, soy sauce, and miso don’t serve as health foods for them. They should also avoid coffee and alcohol as these are also fermented.

Kapha people always have trouble keeping their weight down (their body tends towards anabolism) and are often voluptuous or pear shaped. They have a tendency to have oily skin and hair, and excess fat, hence they should minimize oily or fatty foods. Generally they are easy going, and are often very generous type people. They are the caretaker types in our society. Kapha people will often take care of things, fix things, play “mom” and be there to nurture you. They are good at parenting people. However, when out of balance they can struggle with feeling lethargic in the morning and needing extra coffee to feel mentally alert. They are usually not energetic, "let's get up and go do something" type of people, and prefer "isolating" if given the choice. However, they have excellent stamina when in physical shape.

They walk slowly, hate and often resist exercise, easily develop respiratory problems such as chest colds, or problems with water retention, swollen breasts during PMS, and sometimes produce voluminous quantities of sweat. The extra dampness in their bodies can make their limbs feel heavy, stiff, dull and achy, along with making the palms of their hands damp. This dampness can also cause some types of chronic depression. Nausea is a kapha imbalance associated with extreme dampness and fullness in the digestive tract, stomach and spleen. Some types of edema and damp kinds of asthma are kapha related illnesses. Therefore, the kapha predominate person is most sensitive to damp, as well as cold weather conditions. Late winter and spring are the most aggravating times of the year for them.

In Chinese medicine, Kapha people usually have health problems due to "excess" conditions, along with the tendency to be cold. Their abundant mucus production makes them more susceptible to developing cysts, tumors, uterine fibroids, white thick leukorrhea, sometimes thick cloudy urine, having a sweet sticky taste in the mouth as well as thick saliva, and a greasy white coated tongue. Despite the problems associated with imbalanced kapha, these people always tell me: "I never get sick, but I just don't feel well for some reason."

The kapha person should avoid most dairy products and too many sweet, heavy, gooey foods. Also included in this group for them to avoid is: yogurt, sour cream, cottage cheese, tofu, soy products, winter squashes, sweet potatoes, zucchini, cucumbers, melons, grapefruit, bananas, lemons, pineapple, oranges, and oatmeal.

As you can see from detailed descriptions of the doshas and their characteristics above, patterns of disharmony exist. When vata is in excess in the body, vata related diseases exist such as tissue, blood or plasma deficiency disorders like a scanty menstrual period, osteoarthritis, or degenerative nerve problems. When pitta is excess or disturbed in the body, pitta related health problems occur like sore throats or inflammatory pain, and so on. However, as said earlier in this book, please be aware that despite the constitutional body/mind type, vata people can have pitta imbalances, pitta people can have vata or kapha imbalances and kapha people can have pitta or vata imbalances. For more examples, you can be a predominantly pitta person who temporarily has insomnia that may be a vata type of insomnia (vata imbalance). Then again, it may be a pitta type of insomnia due to an agitated liver. If you are a kapha, you can have either a kapha, pitta, or vata related health problem, but it is more unlikely that you will have a vata related imbalance. It is also important to say again that various manifestations of the same disease exist. There are kapha types of arthritis, vata types, and pitta types. In addition to this, one person can have a mixture of the different types by having two or three doshas out of balance. A kapha – pitta person or just kapha predominate person can have a kapha and pitta related type arthritis at the same time. They might have what they describe as alternating burning and inflammatory type pain, along with a constant dull aching pain that improves with movement. Another example of this mixed symptom pattern, is a person with both a dry hacking cough and a sore throat. Vata is out of balance, evident by the dryness in the cough, and pitta by the inflammation in the throat causing it to be sore. This can get a little complicated when selecting treatments for that individual, and herbs need to be more carefully combined. Herbs and foods, for the latter case, should decrease both dryness and inflammation.

Knowing something about your system, the way it works, and its current state of imbalance is the key to knowing how to treat it when it falls out of balance. Restoring that balance begins with giving it the right foods, the right herbs, natural supplements, lifestyle, exercise for your unique system and/or current medical imbalance.

3

Personalized Nutrition

Nutrition: How Foods Cause and Prevent Disease

I hinted at the beginning of this book, that all foods and herbs have certain energetic and nutritional properties, as well as specific tastes. Some foods are drier than others (diuretic), lighter than others, some heating, some cooling to the body, some increase moisture or water retention, build blood, soften tissue, make muscle contract, and some taste sweet, sour, bitter, etc. Some are higher in B vitamins and some are higher in potassium or vitamin C. Each food, because of its special property, has the ability to reduce the doshas or aggravate them, hence cause disease or restore health! Besides foods containing the obvious substances: vitamins, proteins, fats, carbohydrates, minerals, they also have the qualities of the doshas such as being damp, heavy, light, sticky, sweet, dry, hot, cold, and they have specific obvious tastes.

All in all, there are six main tastes experienced on the tongue from food: sweet, sour, salty, bitter, astringent, and pungent. Sweet substances tend to be heavier, moistening (damp), help build up and lubricate tissue including bone density, strengthen nerve tissue, promote weight gain, etc. Sour things help the body attract and retain moisture and hence increase plasma content, are acidic, increase digestive enzyme activity, are sometimes heating, sometimes not, help tissue relax and become smoother and softer, are higher in vitamin C. Sour substances are excellent for dry, rough skin and constipation! Salty things help the body also retain water and are heating in Ayurveda. (The heating property of salt is why many people want more salt in their cooking during the month of December). Bitter things are catabolic (break down tissue), make tissues contract, tighten muscles, are drying, cold, are higher in B vitamins, etc. Hence bitter foods and substances will aggravate muscle spasms by making them contract! Bitter foods and substances also help fight infection in the body and cool inflammation. (Long term use of bitters on the body, however, are weakening, as they break substances down, not strengthen them. This is one reason why bitter herbs like echinacea should never be used for extended periods of time). Astringent substances are diuretic, light, drying, and contracting. They are excellent for weight loss, and diarrhea. Astringent foods are also hemostatic (stop some types of bleeding). Pungent substances are heating, break up matter, help release some types of stagnation, and improve circulation with their "fire" and "airy" qualities. They move blood and can help dissolve cysts for these reasons, and help break up blood clots and some types of tumors.

For example, apples are light, astringent, sweet, and cooling. When you bite into one, it "crunches," is crispy and feels light. Oatmeal is sweet, heavy, damp, mushy, heating, etc. Bananas, on the other hand, are heavy, damp, sweet, sour, soft, and heating. These heavy damp attributes make them a poor choice for weight loss, but an excellent choice for dry skin. Although bananas and apples have approximately the same number of calories (100 each), you can taste and feel their physical and chemical differences on the body. Lemons, yogurt, vinegar, and pickles are sour and acidic like vitamin C, as well as moistening. They are a poor choice for cases of heartburn, canker sores, and colitis. Seafood is salty, sweet, heavy and heating. Legumes (beans) are astringent, light, drying/diuretic, and cold (except lentils, which are heating). They are a great choice for certain types of edema, diarrhea, and excellent for weight loss. The exception here is tofu, which is a cooling, heavy, damp legume. Its cooling properties are the reason it decreases hot flashes so well, along with other soy products. Yet at the same time, its heavy watery nature makes it a bad choice for a woman that has a thick, white, mucusy cough, or is trying to lose weight. Lettuce, kale and spinach are bitter, airy, catabolic, drying, and cold. This is the reason why they help people lose weight, and help cool inflammation in the body! Garlic is pungent, hot, light, etc.

To experience firsthand the physical and chemical effects of food on the human body, you can spend a week eating popcorn and salads and watch your stools become harder and skin become drier; or spend a week eating nothing but ice cream, yogurt, melons, oranges, spaghetti with tomato sauce, cottage cheese, and grape juice and watch your stools become looser, more watery, and your skin get softer, as well as possibly developing nausea from all this wet, heavy, sweet, rich food! Hence, food affects the disease process very strongly!

If a food has the same qualities of a dosha, then it will increase that dosha and aggravate it. Foods with opposite qualities of that dosha will reduce it and relieve it. Generally, sweet, sour, and salty things reduce vata and are good for vata related diseases because vata tends to be contracted, dry and deficient. Substances with these properties help soften, moisten, build and relax tissue in the body. Sweet, bitter, astringent foods are good for reducing pitta, since pitta is acidic and hot, and they counteract acidity and cool the body (sugar is cooling in its energy and helps hot flashes). Pitta disorders such as many types of skin rashes will benefit from them. Bitter, pungent, astringent substances are good for kapha predominant people and disorders, because substances with these properties help break up mucus, drain dampness, break down tissue/promote catabolism, and promote circulation.

Remember, to reduce an excess dosha in the body to restore balance, foods and substances with the opposite properties must be consumed. If you are a vata predominant person with a vata imbalance, then a vata reducing diet will most likely help reverse the problem you have. If you are a pitta-kapha person with a pitta imbalance, than a pitta-kapha diet will help you with a slight slant towards emphasizing pitta reducing foods that don't aggravate kapha. By the same token, vata predominate people or people with vata imbalances will be aggravated by dry, light, and airy foods such as popcorn, granola, beans, broccoli, cauliflower, cabbage, Brussels sprouts, dried fruits, rye, cornbread, and these foods will often be harder to digest promoting bloating and gas in the digestive tract. These foods are diuretic and not conducive to tissue building. Pitta people or people with pitta imbalances such as inflammatory pain, or acid reflex, should avoid or minimize sour/acidic, fermented and spicy foods as these will more strongly aggravate their already acidic and warm systems; and kapha people or people with kapha medical problems should avoid heavy, damp, sweet, sour, salty, sticky foods as these foods promote water retention, weight gain, and mucus production in the body.

Foods and Their Unique Energetic Properties

Below are some foods listed with their unique energetic properties to give you a clearer picture of these concepts.

Fruits

Apples – sweet, astringent, cooling, drying, light (reduces pitta and kapha, increases vata)

Avocado - sweet, cooling, moistening, oily, heavy (reduces vata and pitta, increases kapha)

Bananas – sweet, sour, warming, moistening, heavy (reduces vata, increases pitta and kapha)

Cantaloupe – sweet, heating, moistening, heavy (reduces vata and pitta, increases kapha)
Cherries – sweet, astringent, sometimes sour, warming, light (reduces vata, pitta, and kapha)
Coconut – sweet, cooling, moistening, oily, heavy (reduces vata and pitta)
Cranberries – sour, heating, drying, light (reduces kapha)
Dates - sweet, astringent, cooling, heavy (reduces vata and pitta)
Figs – sweet, cooling, heavy unless dried figs (reduces vata and pitta)
Grapefruit – sour, cooling, moistening, heavy (reduces vata, increase pitta and kapha)
Grapes – **purple** are sweet, cooling, moistening, heavy (reduces vata and pitta, increases kapha); **green** are sweet, sour, heating, moistening, heavy (reduces vata, increases pitta and kapha)
Lemons/Limes – sour, cooling, moistening, heavy (reduces vata, increases pitta and kapha)
Oranges – sweet, sour, heating, moistening, heavy (reduces vata, can aggravate pitta, increases kapha)
Peaches – sweet, astringent, heating (reduces vata, okay for pitta in moderation, okay for kapha)
Pears – sweet, astringent, cooling, moistening (decreases vata, pitta, kapha)
Pineapple – sweet, sour, heating, moistening, heavy (decrease vata, can aggravate pitta if sour, increases kapha)
Strawberries – sour, cooling, drying, light (decreases kapha, and vata, increases pitta)
Watermelon - sweet, cooling, moistening, heavy (decreases vata and pitta, increases kapha)

Vegetables

Artichokes (globe) – sweet, astringent, heavy, moist, heating (decreases vata and pitta, increases kapha)

Bell peppers – pungent, light, drying, heating (decreases kapha, okay for pitta in moderation, increases vata)

Broccoli – astringent, sweet, cold, light (decreases pitta and kapha, increases vata)

Carrots – pungent, sweet, light, drying, heating (decreases kapha and vata, okay for pitta in moderation)

Cauliflower – astringent, sweet, light, cold (decreases pitta and kapha, increases vata)

Corn on cob – sweet, astringent, light, drying, heating (decreases vata, pitta, and kapha)

Cucumbers - sweet, cooling, heavy (decreases vata and pitta, increases kapha)

Green beans – sweet, stringent, light, cold, drying (decreases vata, pitta, and kapha)

Kale – bitter, light, drying, cold (decreases pitta and kapha, increases vata)

Lettuce – astringent, bitter, light, drying, cold (decreases pitta and kapha, increases vata)

Mushrooms – pungent, light, drying, heating (decreases pitta and kapha, increases vata)

Peas – sweet, astringent, light, drying, cold (decreases pitta and kapha, increases vata)

Potatoes (white) – astringent, light, drying, cold (decreases pitta and kapha, increases vata)

Red radish – pungent, heating, light, drying (decreases kapha and vata, increases pitta)

Tomatoes – sour, heavy, moist, heating (decreases vata, increases pitta and kapha)
Winter squashes – sweet, heavy, moist, cold (decreases vata and pitta, increase kapha)
Zucchini – sweet, pungent, heavy, moist, cold (decreases vata and pitta, increases kapha)

Whole Grains
Buckwheat – pungent, sweet, light, drying, warming (decreases kapha, increases vata and pitta)
Cornmeal – sweet, drying, light, heating (decreases kapha, increases pitta and vata)
Millet – pungent, sweet, drying, light, heating (decreases kapha, increases pitta and vata)
Oats – sweet, heavy, moist, warming (decreases vata and pitta, increase kapha)
Rice - brown – sweet, heavy, moist, warming (decreases vata, increases pitta and kapha); **white** – sweet, heavy, moist, cooling (decreases vata and pitta, increases kapha)
Rye – pungent, sweet, astringent, drying, light, heating (decreases kapha, increases pitta and vata)
Wheat – sweet, heavy, moist, cold (decreases vata and pitta, increases kapha)

Beans (all beans decrease pitta and kapha, but increase vata; tofu and processed soy products decrease vata and pitta, but increase kapha)
Most beans are basically sweet, astringent, light, drying, and cold
Lentils are sweet, astringent, somewhat moist and heating

Tofu and soy foods are sweet, heavy, moist, and cold, unless flavored with soy sauce and spices, which makes them more heating

Dairy

Cheese – sour, salty, fermented, heavy, moist, heating (decreases vata, increases pitta and kapha)

Eggs – whole - sweet, heating, light (decreases vata and kapha, increases pitta); **whites -** sweet, cooling, light (decreases vata, pitta, and kapha)

Ice cream – sweet, heavy, moist, cold (decreases vata and pitta, increase kapha)

Milk – sweet, heavy, moist, cold (decreases vata and pitta, increases kapha)

Ricotta/cottage cheese – sweet, cooling, moist, heavy (decreases vata and pitta, increases kapha)

Sour Cream - sour, fermented, heavy, moist, heating (decreases vata, increases pitta and kapha)

Yogurt – sour, sweet, fermented, heavy, moist, heating (decreases vata, increases pitta and kapha)

Meats (in my opinion, all meats are tridoshic = reduce all three doshas, but seafood aggravates kapha)

Beef – sweet, heavy, moist, heating

Chicken – sweet, astringent, heating

Seafood – sweet, salty, heavy, moist, heating

Venison – light, drying, heating

Nuts (all nuts decrease vata, and increase pitta and kapha)

Most nuts are sweet, heavy, oily, moist, heating

Cooking Oils (all oils decrease vata and increase pitta and kapha)
Canola oil – sweet, cooling
Corn oil – sweet, heating
Olive oil – pungent, heating
Soybean oil – sweet, cooling

Spices – All spices are heating with the exception of dill, mint, fennel, cumin, coriander, saffron, and vanilla. However, some spices are more heating than others such as chili powder being more heating than basil. Garlic is more heating than parsley. Therefore, most spices aggravate pitta, but decrease vata and kapha.

The other interesting fact about Ayurvedic medicine and its perspective on nutrition/food, is that each unique diet or group of foods recommended for the different body types, contain different nutrients or more of some vitamins and minerals than others. This helps that particular body type stay in balance, since that body type has specific nutrient needs that differs from others. For example, the vata recommended diet is naturally higher in vitamin C than any of the other diets, and vatas also have the greatest biological need for this vitamin. The pitta diet is higher in calcium than any other diet, and contains only very low amounts of acidic foods. This is extremely helpful to the pitta person who has a natural biological tendency to be more acidic, put out greater amounts of hydrochloric acid, etc., than most people. Ayurvedic nutrition is a carefully thought-out science and goes well beyond and much deeper than analyzing only proteins, fats, carbohydrates, vitamins and minerals in food content. However, Ayurveda doesn't exclude this type of information either and uses it.

Many times so-called "nutritionists" and "dieticians" miss the boat entirely on the subject of nutrition because they get hung up on proteins, fats, carbohydrates, certain vitamins or nutrients in the foods. They entirely neglect the energetic chemical properties of foods that affect the body's tissues, organs, and their function. An example of this, is an article I read, which told readers to avoid alfalfa sprouts at the salad bar because of their low nutrient value compared to tomatoes. The author of the article, didn't tell the readers that sprouts are excellent for healthy liver function. And the cucumbers that were pooh-poohed for the same reason are excellent for disorders related to excessive dryness, blood and plasma deficiency because of the high water content in them. What's described above in my book, is from a different perspective that most people are unfamiliar with. If you are curious about specific protein, fat, and vitamin value of particular foods, many books on the market exist with material containing this information, and can easily be picked up and read.

What follows are special recommended diets for five of the nine body/mind types (I left out the vata/kapha type because I personally believe this combination type does not exist, and I have not included pitta/vata and kapha/pitta). I also left out the tridoshic type because this person can work on reducing whatever dosha is out of balance at the time and then go back to eating a wide variety of foods when in balance again. Remember, tridoshic people have equal amounts of vata, pitta, and kapha in them). Base your food choices on the appropriate diet for your body type tendencies. This will be a starting point to help restore your balance. Also, be sure to take into account your health problems/imbalances. So for example, if you are a kapha predominant person with a pitta health problem, such as heat or inflammation, avoid hot spices, heating substances, and follow the pitta-kapha recommended diet with an emphasis on pitta reducing foods within that particular diet. However, when selecting the appropriate diet, what feels right to you, is probably pretty correct for you. The food, if very right, will be some of your favorite foods and match your body system. Ayurvedic holds the belief that we are intuitively drawn to substances that help keep us in balance. The information will also make common sense to you and feel intuitively right. Again, if any food on a list gives you gas, diarrhea, heartburn, bloating, nausea, or tastes gross, avoid it and listen to your body. It may not be right for you or your current medical condition. For example, if you are a vata with a pitta imbalance like acid reflex, then sour foods like orange juice and sour cream will probably aggravate your system!

You will also notice that bananas are not recommended for some types of people, since they are damp, heavy, sweet and sour. Many people ask me where do they get their potassium from, then? I tell them there are other sources. One glass of orange juice actually has about 450 mg of potassium in it, roughly the same amount in one banana. Remember, there are many other sources for nutrients that most people aren't aware of, such as kale and collard greens containing large amounts of calcium. In fact, one cup of collards has more calcium than one glass of milk. Okra, broccoli, tofu, carrot juice, blackstrap molasses, and sardines also contain considerable amounts of calcuim. Even vitamin C is found in food sources other than orange juice, such as bell peppers, and tomatoes. Most people assume iron is only found in red meat, but dark leafy greens contain a good supply of it, along with beets, yams, legumes, and purple grapes.

However, I cannot stress enough again, that the most important dietary advice is to eat in line with your genetics and disease tendency. This will help you prevent or minimize the problems that you are most likely to develop as you age. By doing this you will be "outsmarting" your genetics- your body's system, and the way it tends to behave. For example, if your body/genetic type tends to retain fluid, then eating a drier more diuretic diet over one's lifetime, will help minimize the chance of developing serious complicated edema by age 60 or so. If your body tends to over-heat vey quickly (you have a pitta imbalance or pitta type genetics), then eating more cooling foods and avoiding spices over an extended period of time can minimize your chance of developing serious heat related health problems such as high blood pressure or inflammatory pain. Foods such as icecream, sugar, and salads do this. Remember, what's healthy is a relative term- it depends on the individual and medical case. Don't get fooled or sucked in by peer pressure on what's best to eat for your own body!

Diets for Body Type and Disease Tendency

Below are my suggested diets for five of the most commonly seen body/mind types. Keep in mind that not every food listed may be perfect for you. (The foods below help reduce the doshas.):

Vata
(avoid beans, granola, corn chips, dry foods, cruciferous veggies like broccoli, cauliflower, cabbage, kale, Brussels sprouts, peas, living on too many salads)

Whole grains - oatmeal, brown and white rices, whole wheat products
Tofu only. No beans.
Vegetables (primarily cooked) - pumpkin, sweet potatoes/yams, sweet winter squashes, spaghetti squash, tomatoes and sauce, onions, artichokes, carrots, beets, parsnips, okra, green beans, asparagus, yellow summer squashes, zucchini, corn on cob, olives, lettuce, spinach, cucumbers, avocado, plantains
Fruits - grapes, plums, cherries, blueberries, apricots, peaches, pears, melons, dates, figs, coconut, mangoes, pineapple, oranges, bananas, kiwis, lemons, limes, grapefruit **(note: the vata person should also consume plenty of fruit juices regularly)**

Nuts - any
Dairy - milk, cottage cheese, ricotta cheese, ice cream, yogurt, cheese, sour cream, buttermilk
Eggs
Spices – mild strength to spicy
Meats - seafood, dark meat poultry, beef, pork

Vata/Pitta
(avoid super hot spices, granola, beans, dried fruits, raw veggies except salad)

Whole grains - whole wheat products, oatmeal, brown and white rices
Beans – tofu, and soy products only
Vegetables - Sweet winter squashes, sweet tomato sauce, pumpkin, parsnips, spaghetti squash, artichokes, yams, spaghetti squash, carrots, potatoes, onions, bell peppers, mushrooms, cooked broccoli, cooked cauliflower, kale, collards, bok choy, okra, yellow summer squash, zucchini, corn on cob, green beans, peas, spinach, asparagus, lettuce, celery, sprouts, avocado, red radish, black olives.
Fruits – red apples, pears, raisins, oranges, pineapple, green and purple grapes, plums, prunes, cherries, blueberries, apricots, peaches, coconut, dates, figs, cantaloupe, mangoes, bananas, possible kiwis and very sweet lemonade.
Nuts – peanut butter, cashews, macadamia, pistachios
Dairy – milk, cream cheese, cottage cheese, ricotta cheese, sweetened fruity yogurt, mild cheeses, ice cream.
Whole eggs/egg whites
Spices – moderate and medium strength

Meats – poultry, seafood, beef, pork

Pitta
(avoid fermented foods, sour fruits and juices, spicy foods, coffee; this is the one body/genetic type that <u>can</u> really use white sugar)

Whole Grains – whole wheat breads, pasta, pancakes, muffins, oatmeal, white rice, box sweetened cereals
Beans - any (but no soy burgers or veggie mock meats which contain soy sauce, malt)
Vegetables – sweet winter squashes, sweet potatoes/yams, kale, collards, white potatoes, artichokes, mushrooms, cooked onions, sweet red bell peppers, cooked broccoli, cauliflower, cabbage, burdock, Brussels sprouts, peas, asparagus, bok choy, green beans, okra, zucchini, yellow summer squash, corn on cob, spinach, lettuce, celery, sprouts, avocado, cucumbers, coleslaw
100% Sweet Fruits – red sweet apples, pears, grapes, raisins, prunes, plums, cherries, sweetened blueberries, apricots, peaches, melons, dates, coconut, figs, oranges, pineapple, mangoes
Seeds/Nuts - peanut butter/peanuts, sunflower seeds, poppy seeds
Unfermented Sweet Dairy – milk, vanilla ice cream, pudding, ricotta cheese, cream cheese, cottage cheese
Egg Whites
Spices – none except dill, cumin, cilantro, no hot spices
Meats – poultry, seafood, beef, pork

Pitta/Kapha
(avoid hot spices, yogurt, bananas, too much citrus, winter squashes, oatmeal)

Whole grains – wheat products, bread, pasta, bagels, muffins, cornbread, corn grains, white rice, barley, granola, oat bran, dry cereals, corn flakes, popcorn, corn chips, pretzels, wheat crackers
Beans – any legume but no tofu (too damp!)
Vegetables – spaghetti squash, white potatoes, asparagus, bell peppers, burdock, carrots, artichokes, leeks, cooked onions, broccoli, cauliflower, cabbage, Brussels sprouts, kale, collards, corn on cob, yellow summer squashes, green beans, peas, okra, endive, radichio, spinach, lettuce, cucumbers, sprouts.
Fruits – apples, pears, raisins, red grapes, plums, prunes, peaches, apricots, cherries, blueberries, sweetened berries, strawberries, mango, watermelon, honeydew.
Seeds - pumpkin, sunflower
Dairy – skim milk, soymilk, rice milk, vanilla ice cream, mild cheeses
Eggs and Whites
Spices – very mild like parsley, dill, basil, not hot!
Meats – poultry, beef, pork, trout, catfish, venison

Kapha (the pure kapha type with cold and dampness)

Whole grains – corn, buckwheat, millet, rye, amaranth, quinoa, rices, rice cakes, pretzels, crackers, corn chips, popcorn
Beans – any legume but no soy foods
Vegetables – broccoli, cauliflower, cabbage, Brussels sprouts, kale, collards, mustard greens, kohlrabi, daikon and red radish, onions, leeks, garlic, spinach, lettuce, sprouts, green beans, peas, yellow summer squash, corn on cob, spaghetti squash, beets, turnips, carrots, burdock root, endive, radichio
Fruits – apples, pears, raisins, prunes, cherries, berries, cranberries, peaches, apricots, strawberries, dried fruits
Spices – any including hot spices
Meats – white meat poultry, beef, fresh water fish, venison, rabbit, dry meats

4

Demystifying Herbal Medicine

How Herbs Reverse the Disease Process

Just as foods have certain specific tastes and energetic chemical properties, so do herbs, and because of this, they can be the catalysts in your recovery. Herbs can help up build plasma content and in the human body, and also act as diuretics. They can cause muscle tissue to contract or relax, help soften tissue, increase body heat, cause internal coldness, moisten the body and increase fluid retention, and either help promote catabolism (the breakdown of tissue) or anabolism (the build up of tissue). They can build up qi in the body (strength, immunity, and your vitality), or reduce it by weakening you. Additionally, herbs can treat pain, are antibiotic, anti-inflammatory, can nourish tissues, are anti-spasmodic, can lower fevers, and act as a sedative. The main difference between foods and herbs is that the energetic properties in herbs are more concentrated than those in foods. They help get you where you want to go much faster. Technically, your diet should be able to help reverse your condition on its own, but that process might take one to three years. If the illness you have is serious or complicated, then diet alone is not as helpful. It doesn't mean you always have to use herbs to get well either. However, you shouldn't abuse this power and knowledge by ignoring your diet, otherwise the problem you have is more likely to keep resurfacing.

Basically, the six tastes present in food: sweet, salty, sour, bitter, astringent and pungent are also present in herbs. From the Ayurvedic perspective, because of their tastes and energetic properties, herbs will either aggravate the doshas or relieve them.

Generally, pungent, astringent, bitter (warm, dry, and light) herbs reduce kapha related health problems, since they drain dampness (are diuretic), decrease heaviness/mass, circulate blood, break up stagnation and mucus, and tighten tissues by making them contract. Sweet, salty, sour, heavy herbs usually reduce vata in the system since they restore heaviness/build tissue, help build fat, increase blood and plasma, increase moisture in the body, softness, flexibility, and relax tissue. Sweet, bitter, astringent and cold herbs reduce pitta because they reduce heat, stop inflammation, stop infection, and neutralize acid production in the body. The sweet herbs build up tissue and moisten a pitta person, while the bitters cool, dry, are antibiotic, and strongly anti-acid.

Why People Choose the Wrong Herbs

These factors are the main reason why people take an herb for a health problem and it doesn't always work. If you have a medical condition due to too much kapha in your system, or excessive dampness in your tissues causing water retention (edema), then herbs with kapha increasing (damp) properties will aggravate your medical problem. For example, taking the moistening herbs: licorice root and hawthorn berries can cause edema (water retention).

If a person has a vata related health problem and took vata increasing/aggravating herbs, they probably made their problem worse, such as taking sage and mullein leaf for a dry cough or dry respiratory problem (sage and mullein are drying type herbs). There are also several different types of insomnia. If you take an herb such as chamomile or skullcap, but the type and cause of your insomnia is high/excess vata (nerve tissue deficiency or weakness), then neither of those herbs is going to work, although they have sedative properties and are considered nervine herbs. Chamomile and skullcap increase vata in the body because they are bitter herbs, and bitters contain air and ether qualities. As you learned, bitters or airy substances break down tissue, including nerve tissue, and promote catabolism. This is where the statement "he/she has weak nerves" comes from.

If you have insomnia and are a pitta person, or have a current pitta imbalance with a lot of heat, taking valerian (a known herbal sedative), will aggravate your system because the energetics of the herb are antagonistic to pitta or "heating." Valerian's warming and pungent properties can also aggravate inflammatory type pain, or cause headaches if you have them.

So just because an herb is said to relieve a particular medical condition, doesn't mean it necessarily will. This is the single biggest reason most people take the wrong herbs. They look up a particular herb in a book and read what the herb does, or under what conditions or diseases it is listed. Herbology is much more complicated than that. To treat illness, you must be specific in your approach. One must take into consideration the nature of his/her system, (biological tendencies/body type), the current state of imbalance or aggravated dosha(s), take the specific symptoms into consideration, and the energetic properties of the herbs you are considering to use. A good practitioner helping you will also take your prescription drugs (if you are on any) into consideration to make sure no harmful interactions occur. Without doing any of the above, the program you follow is likely to be fruitless.

Specific Properties of Herbs

I have listed below a very short list of some of the hundreds of herbs used, their energetic properties, and their relationship to the doshas. To find out exactly what the herbs do and what they are specifically used for, consult a good herbal reference book.

Vata reducing/balancing herbs (reduce dryness, tissue deficiency)

Amalaki – heavy, sour, moistening, cooling (aggravates pitta, increase kapha)

Angelica– heating, sweet, pungent (aggravates pitta, but also reduces kapha)

Ashwagandha– heating, heavy, sweet, moistening (aggravates pitta, increases kapha)

Astragalus root – warm, sweet, moistening (also reduces pitta mildly, but can aggravate if heat present)

Bala – sweet, cooling, heavy, moistening (also reduces pitta, increases kapha)

Citrus peel – warm, bitter (also reduces kapha and pitta mildly)

Comfrey – cooling, heavy, moistening, softening (also reduces pitta, increases kapha)

Codonopsis – neutral, sweet, moistening, heavy (also reduces pitta, increases kapha)

Fennel - cooling, heavy, sweet, moistening (also reduces pitta, increases kapha)

Fo-ti (Ho-Shou-Wu) - cooling, heavy, moistening (also reduces pitta, increase kapha)

Ginseng – heating , heavy, sweet, pungent (aggravates pitta, increases kapha)

Hawthorn Berries – sour, sweet, warming, heavy (aggravates pitta, increases kapha)

Irish moss – salty, sweet, astringent, heating, heavy, moistening (aggravates pitta, increases kapha)

Licorice – cooling, sweet, heavy, moistening, bitter (also reduces pitta, increases kapha)

Longan fruit – warm, sweet (may reduce pitta somewhat if not overheated, increases kapha)

Lycium fruit – neutral, sweet (also reduces pitta, increases kapha)

Rehmannia root (cooked) – warm, sweet, moistening, heavy (increases kapha) (raw) - cooling, sweet, moistening, heavy (also reduces Pitta, increases kapha)

Rosehips – sour, cooling (aggravates pitta, increases kapha)

Saw palmetto – sweet, pungent, heating (aggravates pitta)

Schizandra fruit – warm, sour, moistening, heavy (aggravates pitta, increases kapha)

Shatavari – cooling, sweet, heavy, moistening, bitter (also reduces pitta, increases kapha)

Slippery Elm – sweet, cooling, heavy, moistening (also reduces pitta, increases kapha)

Valerian – pungent, sweet, astringent, bitter, heating (aggravates pitta)

Wild yam – cooling, sweet, moistening, heavy (also reduces pitta, increases kapha)

Pitta reducing/balancing herbs (reduce acidity and heat)

Aloe Vera – bitter, drying, light, cold (also reduces kapha, increases vata)

Bala – sweet cooling, heavy, moistening (also reduces vata, increases kapha)

Bhumy amalaki – cold, bitter, drying, light (also reduces kapha, increases vata)

Brahmi – bitter, cold, sweet (also reduces vata and kapha)

Bupleurum – bitter, cooling, slightly spicy, drying (also reduces kapha, increases vata)
Burdock root – bitter, pungent, cooling (also reduces kapha, increases vata)
Catnip – pungent, cooling, (also reduces kapha, increases vata)
Chrysanthemum – cooling, bitter, sweet, pungent (also reduces kapha, increases vata)
Cumin – pungent, bitter, cooling (also reduces vata and kapha)
Dandelion – bitter, cold, drying, light (also reduces kapha, increases vata)
Echinacea – cooling, bitter, pungent (also reduces kapha, increases vata)
Guduchi – bitter, warm, sweet (also reduces kapha, increases vata)
Hops – bitter, pungent, cooling (also reduces kapha, increases vata)
Jujube – sweet, neutral (also reduces vata, increases kapha)
Lemongrass – bitter, pungent, cooling, light (also reduces kapha, increases vata)
Licorice – cooling, sweet, heavy, moistening, bitter (also reduces vata, increases kapha)
Marshmallow – cold, sweet, heavy, moistening (also reduces vata, increases kapha)
Peppermint – cold, bitter, drying, light, stimulating (also reduces kapha, increases vata)

Punarnava – bitter, cold, pungent (also reduces kapha, increases vata)
Red Clover – cold, bitter, light, drying (also reduces kapha, increases vata)
Red Raspberry Leaf – cold, astringent, light, drying (also reduces kapha, increases vata)
Skullcap – bitter, cooling, light (also reduces kapha, increases vata)
Shatavari – cooling, sweet, heavy, moistening, bitter (also reduces vata, increases kapha)
Solomon's seal – sweet, cooling, moistening (also reduces vata, increases kapha)
Turmeric – bitter, heating, light, drying, pungent (also reduces kapha, increases vata)

Kapha reducing/balancing herbs (reduce dampness, congestion)

Ashoka – astringent, pungent, cold, sweet (also reduces pitta, increases vata)
Atractylodes - warm, spicy, bitter, drying (aggravates pitta, increases vata)
Black pepper – heating, pungent (aggravates pitta)
Cayenne – heating, pungent, light (aggravates pitta)
Chamomile - cold, bitter and pungent, drying, sedative (also reduces pitta, increases vata)
Cloves – heating, pungent (aggravates pitta)

Crampbark – bitter, astringent, heating (aggravates pitta)
Elecampane – pungent, bitter, heating, light, drying (aggravates pitta)
Eucalyptus – heating, pungent (aggravates pitta)
Garlic – warming, pungent (aggravates pitta)
Ginger – heating, pungent, sweet (aggravates pitta)
Guggul – bitter, pungent, astringent heating (aggravates pitta)
Juniper Berries – pungent, bitter, sweet, heating (increases pitta)
Magnolia bark – warm, spicy, drying (aggravates pitta)
Manjistha – bitter, sweet, cold, pungent (also reduces pitta, aggravates vata)
Parsley – heating, drying, light, pungent, diuretic (aggravates vata)
Pippali – hot, pungent (aggravates pitta)
Sage – pungent, bitter, astringent, heating, light, drying (aggravates pitta)
Saussurea root – warm, spicy, bitter, sweet (aggravates pitta)
Shilajit – pungent, bitter, warm (aggravates vata and pitta)
St. John's Wort – bitter, pungent, cooling, light (also reduces pitta, increases vata)
Thyme – warming, pungent (increases pitta)
Turmeric – warming, bitter, pungent, light, drying (also reduces pitta, increases vata)
Uva Ursi – cooling, bitter, drying, astringent, diuretic (also reduces pitta, aggravates vata)
Vasaka/vasa – bitter, warm (can aggravate pitta, increases vata)

Diagnosing Patterns of Disharmony in Your Body

Knowing how your body works (your body type) is a great asset, because you can almost predict how you will react to an herb before you even take it. That is the beauty of Ayurveda, as a medical system. However, sometimes you may want to treat an illness with herbs by simply treating its pattern of disharmony as Chinese medicine does. What I mean by this, is that if you know you have a problem related to coldness in your system, you may want to try including herbs and foods that dispel coldness. If the problem seems to be caused by excessive dampness, then foods and herbs that have a drying effect on the body will help you. If the pattern is clearly one due to excess fire or heat, cooling foods and herbs will help, and so on. Windy/deficient states will diminish by taking heavier foods and herbs. Dry states are relieved over time by substances with moistening properties. Damp and cold conditions will need both dry and warming herbs to dispel them.

Below are several patterns of disharmony and their symptoms. In Chinese medicine they are called "evils" that can permeate the body:

Dampness manifests in the system sometimes as nausea/lack of appetite, sticky saliva in mouth, lack of the ability to taste one's food, sometimes vomiting, desire to sleep long hours, excess weight gain, loose stools, or diarrhea, stiffness, heaviness, water retention, moist palms, damp skin, thick abundant saliva, a white greasy tongue coating, and when a person feels uncomfortable in humidity. In Ayurveda, although anyone can develop a damp condition, kapha predominant type people are the most susceptible to developing it than any other body type. Some types of edema, and heavy menstrual bleeding are damp related medical problems. Also, some types of asthma and allergies can be a result of this condition.

Excess heat becomes evident when a person feels uncomfortable in hot weather, sweats easily in heat, has a very red tongue, sometimes a rapid pulse, dry tongue or red tongue with yellow fur, sometimes a huge appetite, excessive thirst, hot flashes, possible high fevers, dark yellow colored urine, very warm hands and feet, and sometimes a red face. The pulse may feel rapid. If severe enough or lasting long enough, heat can sometimes dry up the fluids in the body causing constipation, scanty urine or dry skin. In Ayurveda pitta-predominate people are most likely to suffer from heat-related problems. Some heat-related medical problems include: rosacea, psoriasis, inflammatory type arthritic pain, most infections, and hot flashes, as already mentioned above.

Cold conditions cause these types of symptoms to develop: cold hands and feet, frequent and clear urination, aversion to cold weather, lack of thirst and possibly little appetite, a pale colored tongue, pale face, sometimes muscle spasms/cramps (since cold causes muscle tissues to contract), sometimes a slow pulse rate, and the desire to sleep curled up in a ball.

Dry states cause dry cracked skin, dry hair, dandruff/dry scalp, dry mouth and tongue, a parched throat, dry cough with no sputum, constipation, vaginal itching with dryness, sometimes lack of sweat in heat, sometimes cracking in the spine and joints, and thirst. As mentioned before, vata imbalances are often because of excess dryness in the body. Some health problems caused in part from excessive dryness include: some types of female hair loss, osteoarthritis, a scanty mentrual period, and some types of allergies and asthma.

Windy states can cause tremors in the hands and tongue, dizziness, light headedness, some kinds spasms, ringing in the ears, shaking of the head, some types of hyperactivity. Wind can cause pain to migrate in the body, shift from one location to the next. Its symptoms may appear suddenly and come and go. In Ayurveda, vata people are more likely to develop health problems as a result of this type of imbalance in the body.

For more specific examples of these principles and how they work, nausea is sometimes related to, but not in all cases, too much dampness and sometimes cold in the stomach or spleen. In Ayurveda, nausea is usually a sign of localized high kapha in the stomach that means too much dampness and/or cold putting out the digestive fire. Many people experience it after eating a heavy Thanksgiving meal. Therefore, herbs that are light, warming, and pungent may help reverse this problem. Ginger is a common remedy used for this condition because it contains those properties. Basically, anything mildly spicy and light will help dispel nausea, including light spicy food in small amounts. Spicy Mexican bean dishes, salads, apples, coffee, and cranberry juice may be appropriate foods in this case. Sometimes the lack of gastric enzymes or acidity can cause food to stagnate and cause nausea. In this case, slightly sour foods and beverages may help like grapefruit, or lemon in water.

If you have a dry mouth and throat during a cold virus you developed, then more juicy juices and herbs with moistening properties will help. Drinking plenty of orange, coconut, grape and pineapple juice helps increase the plasma content in the body and thus alleviate dryness. The herb licorice root is one herb out of many that also do this. Since licorice root is cooling as well as moistening, it is a good choice for dry and inflamed sore throat. Solomon's seal, wild yam and rehmannia root all do the same thing. They restore yin to the body. Because they are basically moistening cool herbs, they will work best on dry conditions with heat. Dry conditions with cold, will need both demulcent, moistening herbs and heating spices to make the formula overall more warming.

A heat disharmony, evident by a red tongue, bloodshot or red eyes, aversion to hot weather, a red face, excessive thirst, and possibly rapid pulse, will benefit from cooling herbs. A chronic condition of severe sore throats, tonsil infections, or high fevers along with these symptoms, clearly indicates a heat pattern. If there is also dampness associated with a heat pattern, then cooling dry herbs are a good choice. If dryness is evident with the heat, then cool moist herbs are the better choice. By applying these principles to natural healing, you are being specific in your treatment approach and are more likely to get the results you so much desire!

In addition to the above-described Chinese patterns of disharmony, I would like to mention three other patterns: qi deficiency, excess qi states, and blood deficiency. All three conditions can be treated by a change in diet, lifestyle, and herbal medicine. I mentioned earlier in this book that vata types tend to develop qi and blood deficiency conditions and kapha types are more prone to excess qi conditions. Generally, qi is considered the vitality, energy force, or essence of life and the body. When someone's organs or body has good abundant qi, we say the organs are strong, the body and immune system are strong, and the person's energy and stamina are excellent!

Deficiency states are associated with a frail, weak physical appearance, weight loss, perhaps emaciation, deficient blood as in certain types of anemic conditions, and in women, a scanty menstrual flow that lasts only two-three days. Other symptoms include, male impotence, deficient fluids/plasma causing a dry state in the body, a lack of vitality and vigor, visually seeing spots before the eyes, fatigue, certain types of insomnia due to deficiency of nerve tissue, and too much lightness in the body. Deficiency of blood in the heart can cause heart palpitations and anxiety and insomnia as well. Some, but not all types of numbness and tingling in the fingers are due to a weak nervous system (nerves not firing properly), or deficient liver blood. Both deficient blood and plasma can cause dizziness in the person. The person's health is in a wasting state in which they may have no muscular strength. Their voice may sound frail, quiet. Their nature is passive. The pulse is weak, deficient, sometimes thready. In Ayurvedic medicine, we say the seven tissues of the body are in a deficient state (plasma, blood, muscle, fat, bone, marrow, and reproductive tissue), and vata predominate people are more likely to develop these type of problems.

Qi deficiency states usually respond to heavy nourishing herbs and foods such as herbs called "qi tonics." Many of the vata reducing herbs fall into this category and can be used. Ginseng, fo-ti, rehmannia root, licorice root, shatavari, bala, amalaki, chywan prash (Ayurvedic nourishing vata formula), Irish moss, lycium fruit, astragalus, wild yam, jujube, codonopsis, Solomon's seal, and ashwagandha are considered qi tonics.

Excess conditions are the opposite: the person appears to have an abundance of the seven main tissues of the body. They appear robust/strong and overweight, they may have much internal dampness and mucus/congestion in their body. They have a firm handshake. Emotionally they may have tendencies towards lethargy and muddled thinking, as the nerves become dulled. They may feel fatigued, not because of malnutrition, but because of excess dampness/fluid pulling them down and making them feel too grounded. Excess states can cause excess discharges like heavy thick mucus, heavy menstrual bleeding, profuse ear wax and snot, lots of mucus in the cornea of the eyes, very thick oily stools. The person with an excess condition will usually have a distinct gait such as a heavy ponderous one. Their voice may sound slow and heavy or rumbling. The breathing is often heavy and forceful as you can hear it. They may or may not snore. The skin is thick with ample fat below its surface. The illnesses of excess qi are often kapha disorders: sometimes benign cysts and tumors, obesity, damp oily skin. This type of condition responds favorably to kapha reducing herbs and foods such as light, bitter and pungent ones.

Blood deficiency conditions are evident by these symptoms: pale tongue and face, dizziness, seeing spots before the eyes, sometimes dry skin and hair, and if you are female, a scanty menstrual period. In Ayurveda, a scanty menstrual period is a sign of a vata imbalance. A rich nutritive and moistening diet helps reverse this condition with plenty of blood and moisture building herbs. Some food examples are: iron tablets themselves, liver tablets, red meat, seafood, sweet potatoes, winter squashes, cucumbers, zucchini, citrus juices/fruits such as oranges, pineapple, kiwi, bananas, dates, figs, melons, purple grapes, coconut, plums, tomatoes/sauce, artichokes, yogurt, milk, cottage cheese, spinach, beets, brown rice, oatmeal, nuts.

Do keep in mind that people can have mixed states of disharmony, as in Chinese medicine, or dual doshic imbalances, as in Ayurvedic medicine. A person can have both vata and pitta out of balance simultaneously. In Chinese medicine a vata-pitta imbalance might be described as a kidney yang deficiency (a cold pattern weakening and affecting the kidneys), blood deficiency and/or dryness, a qi deficiency case (general weakening of vitality and strength), and liver invading the spleen (a digestive disturbance related to the liver), depending on which symptoms and patterns of disharmony are present at the time. Kidney yang deficiency, blood deficiency, qi deficiency, and liver-spleen deficiency might display the symptoms of coldness in the body, frequent urination, lower back pain, scanty menstrual period, pale skin and pale tongue, slow and weak pulse, chronic fatigue, hair loss, dry nostrils, constipation, irritability, bloating/gas, tenderness/soreness over the liver area of the body, etc. All those symptoms describe vata and pitta traits. More complex cases involve having vata, pitta, and kapha (tridoshic) imbalances at once. When this occurs, the combination of herbs requires more skill and knowledge.

For example, if a person has a hot dry pattern, then herbs such as fo-ti, shatavari, and licorice root will be helpful to include in a formula since these are cool moist herbs. If they have a damp heat problem, then drying and cooling herbs such as punarnava, dandelion, manjistha, aloe vera, peppermint, or chrysanthemum are more appropriate. Suppose the individual has a deficient condition, a dry pattern, a wind pattern, and a cold intolerance. They have symptoms of weakness, fatigue/no stamina, insomnia, a pale tongue with a tremor (wind invasion/nervous system imbalance, and cold or blood deficiency), a very thin, emaciated appearance, muscle spasms, stiffness and pain in the legs that worsens in the winter and fall (cold/dry climates), a dry mouth, dry peeling skin on the hands and constipation. All these symptoms describe a vata disharmony pattern in Ayurveda. I would probably recommend a diet that dispels coldness, dryness, and one that is heavier, moistening, predominantly cooked, and nourishing to the body and nerves, such as a vata decreasing diet in this case. If there are blood deficiency symptoms, then blood increasing herbs, and a vata decreasing diet are definitely needed. For constipation I would recommend triphala and castor oil in orange juice, or maybe licorice root with a bit of ginger added to it. If the person took warm milk (milk has moistening properties), I would have them add a bit of castor oil and cinnamon or ginger to both warm the cold milk and make it more laxative. Cinnamon and ginger increases peristaltic action from my experience. Triphala is somewhat sour and moistens the intestines and colon, is laxative. Also, taking the Indian herb amalaki or the western herb hawthorn berries would help decrease the dryness in the system as these herbs are also sour and promote fluid retention. Drinking plenty of fruit juices would also be recommended to help increase this person's plasma content, and help restore some of the body's moisture more easily than just drinking water. I would consider using angelica, ginger, and guggul with marshmallow root to help with this type of pain and stiffness. This type of pain, in most cases is usually due to dryness, tightness or contraction of the muscles, impeded circulation/stagnation, cold, and a general weakness of the body. Angelica, ginger, and guggul are heating, increase blood circulation, and counteract this type of pain while marshmallow is cooling, heavy and moistening, and also considered an energy/qi tonic (strengthening to the body).

There are many excellent Chinese, Western and Indian formulas, depending on the case. For the case just mentioned, ones that contain a combination of tonics such as ginseng, ho-shou-wu, shatavari, marshmallow, Solomon's seal, rehmannia, or licorice root, along with warming, circulating herbs that help relieve this type of pain or spasms such as frankincense, cinnamon, ginger, gastrodia, or corydalis, would be possible choices. Vitamin C would also help this person's condition, since it is sour, helps relax and moisten tissue, and is heating. Ashwagandha (an Indian herb) could be used also, since it is a warming qi tonic and used for wasting conditions. Ashwagandha also helps build up nerve tissue. It is considered a heavy herb. It could be combined with shatavari, fo-ti, or rehamnnia (qi, blood, and moistening tonics), saussurea, angelica, ginger, and cinnamon. For this type of deficiency insomnia, any of the above tonics: ginseng, shatavari, marshmallow root, ho-shou-wu, rehamnnia, licorice root, and ashwagandha will help build up the nervous tissue. In addition to those, the person could try herbs that both sedate the nerves and relax muscle spasms such as taking a combination of valerian, jatamansi, and nutmeg at bedtime. Slippery elm, vamsha rochana, ho-shou-wu, rehamnnia, shatavari, and licorice root all help the dryness he/she is experiencing, strengthen the entire body, and boost energy, but since they are cold herbs you might need to add ginger, citrus peel, and cinnamon. The possible herb formula combinations are endless, as long as the formula is overall moistening, tonifying, warming, blood circulating, antispasmodic, and overall vata decreasing. A nice external form of treatment could be added to this program, such as warm hot baths and warm heavy oils applied on the skin. Some good heavy rich oils are sesame oil, almond oil, or an ashwagandha and bala oil.

Herbs for the Eight Major Patterns of Disharmony (NOTE: Please research these first before using, since each herb does something different in the body. Example: Peppermint relieves heat as well as dampness, and is mildly stimulating. It would be a poor choice for a cold dry deficient condition. The same for manjistha. Its nature is not just cooling, but drying as well.)

Dry states – Moistening herbs: slippery elm, fo-ti, shatavari, licorice root, ashwagandha, bala, Solomon's seal, amalaki, rehmannia root, vamsha rochana, marshmallow, jujube, codonopsis, hawthorn berries

Damp patterns – Drying herbs: dandelion, parsley, burdock root, red clover, turmeric, elecampane, sage, fenugreek, vasaka, aloe vera, bayberry bark, uva ursi, shilajit, chamomile, peppermint, manjistha, musta, agrimony

Heat patterns – Cooling herbs: peppermint, lemon balm, chrysanthemum, lemongrass, red clover, aloe vera, sandalwood, bala, marshmallow root, fo-ti, shatavari, licorice root, bala, Solomon's seal, fennel, cumin, coriander, rehmannia root, wild yam, codonopsis, echinacea, chamomile

Cold patterns – Warming herbs: cinnamon, orange peel, sage, basil, garlic, cayenne, clove, turmeric, ginger, parsley, sea salt, Irish moss, kelp, ashwagandha, American ginseng, black pepper, angelica, cardamom, eucommia bark, pippali, hingwastak, guggul, juniper berries, crampbark, thyme, shilajit.

Wind states – Heavy herbs: ashwagandha, ginseng, amalaki, shatavari, marshmallow, root, slippery elm, fo-ti, Solomon's seal, kapikacchu, licorice root, rehmannia root, bala, vamsha rochana, wild yam

Deficient states – Tonic herbs - ashwagandha, shatavari, Solomon's seal, astragalus, fo-ti, licorice root, ginseng, rehmannia root, wild yam, kapikacchu, saw palmetto, codonopsis, lycium fruit, jujube, slippery elm, hawthorn berries amalaki, chywan prash, bala, marshmallow, Irish moss, longan berries

Excess states – Reducing herbs - red raspberry leaf, lemongrass, lemon balm, dandelion, burdock root, chrysanthemum, garlic, bhumy amalaki, neem, turmeric, parsley, red clover, yellow dock, aloe vera, ginger, catnip, peppermint, skullcap, trikatu, pippali, elecampane, sage, bayberry, wild cherry bark, cinnamon, black pepper, cayenne, guggul

Blood deficiency - Blood building herbs - ho-shou-wu, rehmannia root, lycium fruit, licorice root, amalaki, Solomon's seal, shatavari, slippery elm, hawthorn berries.

The Different Uses of Herbs

As already hinted above, one herb can also have many different uses. For example, aloe vera gel is traditionally used in Ayurveda both internally and externally. Aloe vera reduces pitta and kapha doshas as it helps break down tissue, drains dampness, as well as cools inflammation. It is a cold, dry, and bitter herb that alleviates hot, damp conditions. (Pitta dosha is hot and Kapha dosha creates dampness.) Topically, it is used for burns on the skin. Internally, it may be prescribed for an infectious pitta condition (aloe is a mild antibiotic, a blood cleanser, clears heat), hot flashes, liver problems, fevers, inflammatory types of pain, kapha type fatigue due to a condition of excess, and lethargy, etc. It is also slightly laxative, although its long term effect on the body is drying. Its cold, bitter, light, and dry nature make it very aggravating to vata and vata imbalances, or cold and/or dry patterns of disharmony.

Ginger root has many different uses as well. This pungent, heating, light herb alleviates kapha dosha because its properties help break up congestion, warm the body, promote circulation, and raise metabolism. It is excellent for treating coughs with heavy mucus, and helps counteract nausea. Ginger's properties are slightly stimulating so kapha people find that it helps decrease the lethargy they frequently experience, in addition to a kapha reducing diet of lighter, dry foods, and a good cup of strong coffee! Conditions of cold in the body respond well to this herb since it is so heating. Ginger is most aggravating to pitta because of its hot pungent properties, and hence will aggravate a condition of colitis, heartburn, diarrhea, or burning inflammatory type pain in the body.

Licorice root as stated above is cooling, heavy, moistening, and sweet. These properties make it balancing to both vata and pitta conditions, therefore helping dry lungs and sinus passages as well as sore throats and inflammation. Its natural sweetness makes it ideal for helping control pitta and vata related blood sugar disorders. The heaviness and sweetness also promote the growth of tissue and therefore it aggravates kapha people and kapha related health problems. It will promote weight gain and in extreme cases when used extensively, promote nausea due to its heaviness. In kapha people with congestive heart failure, hypertension, or edema, it is very dangerous because of its ability to promote water retention. However, licorice will reduce pitta or yang type hypertension. Licorice is also considered an immune and adrenal tonic for vata and pitta people and will increase stamina and strength in these people.

We all know peppermint to be cooling. So this herb is an excellent choice for hot flashes. However, peppermint is drying, bitter, light and a bit stimulating which makes it vata aggravating. Its airy and stimulating properties on the nervous system, make it an excellent herb choice for kapha types. Its bitter, cooling properties are helpful for liver caused headaches. Peppermint also has a slight bronchidilating effect on the respiratory passages, so it can help open breathing passages. As an anti-acid, it can be used in formulas for heartburn. It alleviates conditions of damp heat in the body.

Another important thing you need to know when choosing herbs for illness, is that it is important to choose an herb that not only does what you want (heats, cools, dries, strengthens, etc.), but also goes directly to the area of the body that needs it. Certain herbs are intended to be used specifically for certain purposes. They have a special affinity for certain organs or areas of the body. For example, astragalus root is often used as a tonic for the lungs and spleen and treats disorders there. Licorice root, eucalyptus, elecampane, bayberry bark, wild cherry bark, and bala have that affinity for the lungs also. However, they all have different properties, so you need to check their properties and decide which ones to use under what conditions. Astragalus and licorice are more moistening and also considered to be qi tonics. They will help breathing problems due to internal dryness and/or wasting states, although licorice is much more moistening. Bayberry and elecampane are drying, and help decrease dampness in the lungs and sinuses. They will benefit damp types of asthma.

For another example, valerian and jatamansi are known sedatives, or muscle relaxants. They affect the nervous system and go directly to it. Valerian is warming, jatamansi is cooling and heavy. Catnip and skullcap also go directly to the nervous system, but their properties are different than those of valerian; both are bitter and light herbs. They will affect the nervous system differently in different people and different cases. Since they are lighter and bitter herbs, they often benefit kapha or kapha-pitta type of insomnia which do not need the heaviness and grounding of other herbs to correct it. Their bitterness, as well as sedative properties, makes them nice choices for insomnia caused by an agitated liver, especially in heavier body types. Bitter herbs help stimulate healthy liver qi movement.

Herbal Strength

One last secret I will share with you on the topic of herbal medicine: herbs all have various degrees of strength or what I call potency. For example, although both parsley and uva ursi are both diuretics that reduce kapha in the body, uva ursi is much stronger. Although chamomile and skullcap are sedatives for pitta and kapha imbalances, skullcap is stronger. That doesn't mean you should automatically take the stronger herb. In some cases that could be beneficial and in some cases detrimental. Herbology can be complicated and requires some skill and education. You can also combine herbs with each other to augment their effects, or help lessen the effect of each other. For example, the cold properties of the herb licorice can be slightly offset or minimized by combining cinnamon with it. The heat of ginger can be offset by adding peppermint or licorice to it.

Advice Before Self–Medicating With Herbs (Please read this!)

It is a good idea to thoroughly research any of the herbs or natural substances you decide to take. Just because herbs are natural doesn't mean they are safe. Too often people ignore negative symptoms. If you do find yourself experiencing anything abnormal or unpleasant, discontinue their use immediately. It may mean that the herb or formula is not right for your system and/or medical condition, the dosage is too strong for you, or that your body is very sensitive and/or your case more complicated. In most cases, when people experience side affects, it usually is because they took the wrong herb for their body type/system and their medical condition. When people use the appropriate herbs, the risk of potential side effects diminishes. Also, herbs should not be used long term, as one's condition changes, and therefore side effects can result. For example, if a person has a mild heat imbalance, as in the case of hot flashes, staying on cooling herbs long term not only will diminish the hot flashes, but also can cause a cold condition leading to new health problems.

I have also met many people who are terrified in general to use herbs, and experienced psychosomatic effects when taking them such as anxiety, heart palpitations, etc. This always amazes me because prescription drugs are far more dangerous and concentrated. Did you know that the eighth cause of death in the United States is from side effects of prescription drugs? Far more people have died from taking prescription drugs than herbs. Herbs can hurt you, but it just takes a much longer period of time at higher doses.

In addition to this, Ayurvedic and Chinese medicine have an entirely different view and approach on herbology than Western medicine. As I already pointed out earlier in this book, where Western medicine may prescribe the same drug for everyone based on what it does in terms of treating a particular disease, Ayurvedic medicine makes a differentiation between people's different body systems, different causes or variations of common medical problems, and how the herb will interact, as well as taking into account, besides its function, an herb's energetic properties (cold, hot, drying, moistening, acidic, building, depleting, etc.). This type of deeper understanding is crucial to getting effective results in the treatment of disease. Chinese medicine will also look and determine if the patient needs a cooling or heating, drying, or moistening herb formula based on their specific symptoms.

When in doubt about making choices over which herbs to use, consult a certified and reputable Ayurvedic or Chinese practitioner for the best care, and always exercise caution and intuition. The majority of these people are highly skilled herbalists, and Ayurvedic practitioners are also skilled nutritionists, having studied both for years, not one weekend seminar or month course. General schooling requirements for these fields are 3 to 5 years. Also, be sure to ask to see certifications when choosing a natural health care practitioner, and ask how long it took to receive those certificates. Some claim to be knowledgeable in natural medicine without ever having completed years of schooling for it. They get suggestions from a few weekend seminars, or only from the product information that the companies send them. Many individuals are practicing holistic medicine without any real credentials, to keep up with the growing interest, and to compete with other practitioners whom they see as their new competitors. Currently, in the US, there is no law enforcement regulating this practice. This is very dangerous! As even garlic or ginseng supplements prescribed for the wrong patient could exacerbate or cause hypertension! Many people, unfortunately, never even question the credentials of their physicians.

I have seen many patients in my office hurt in this way without even knowing it. One 33-year-old man in particular that I remember, had inflammatory type pain in which his health care provider prescribed a combination of valerian and barbiturates. A dangerous combination, as both have sedative properties. Also, valerian aggravates and worsens inflammation in the body as it is a heating herb.

In another case, I saw a man in his late fifties. His physician had prescribed golden seal in large doses of about 6 capsules a day for a mild prostrate infection, but suggested that he also stay on the herb indefinitely to prevent the reoccurrence of another infection. Golden seal is a very strong cold, bitter, drying, antibiotic herb that when used over a period of time, can cause muscle contractions, spasms, tightness, dryness, hyperactivity, heart palpitations, etc., especially in vata predominant/thin-gaunt people. By the time this man came to see me in my office, he had classic high vata imbalances: tremors in his hands, impotence, back muscle spasms, leg cramps, hair loss, insomnia, heart palpitations, weight loss, and a diminished immune system with allergies to dry airborne particles, dust and smoke. He had also gone to a Western immunologist, after developing these symptoms, who advised him to abstain from dairy products, sugars, sweet juices, soda, wheat breads, and citrus fruits; the very foods that would have helped reversed his problems. This man's health was deteriorating rapidly. The physician and immunologist did not account for his thin frail body type, and the strength, or dosage of the herbs, nor the proper length of time in which to take them. When this man came to see me, he was afraid to take my advice at this point because he had gotten so much bad information.

It is important never to blindly follow another person's recommendations or worship any health care professional. People can make mistakes or misjudgments, especially if they lack inadequate schooling. I always tell my patients to feel free to ask questions. Also, if you are pregnant, you should further research any of the herbs you are taking because some of them are contraindicated when pregnant. If you have any heart problems or any other potentially life threatening illnesses, please consult your practitioner before undertaking some of the suggestions in this book. Use common sense and listen to your body! Avoid strong exercise or exercise cautiously in weather conditions of extreme heat and remember to hydrate yourself adequately beforehand, during, and after the duration exercise.

Many herbs can safely be combined with prescriptions, however there are some that can not. If you are currently taking prescription drugs, you must be careful. You do not want to be taking herbal painkillers or sedatives if you are also on prescription drugs that are designed to do the same thing. The same common sense should be applied if you are on blood thinners for a heart condition, or simply aspirin, fatty acids, or extra vitamin E. You do not want to be taking bitter herbs in combination with these substances, as they are also anti-coagulants. Again, consult a certified and qualified professional practitioner of natural medicine. Be sure to keep up your appointments.

When I had a woman with hypertension who wanted to try strictly natural methods, I had her have her blood pressure monitored frequently by her physician or nurse. Your physician may want to reduce the dosage of the prescription you are taking if the natural medicines and lifestyle changes are actually working for you. I have had many people taper off their prescriptions, in conjunction with supervision from their medical doctor, as their condition began to recede. You can develop a harmonious relationship with your Western physician in this way. Why not have medical help from the best of both worlds: conventional western medicine and natural medicine?

Last, because people are indeed different from one another physiologically, when making food and herb choices within the recommendations in this book for a specific medical condition, please listen to your body. If there are one or several foods or herbs that create discomfort, give you gas, etc., don't take them. However, beware that many of the herbs are strong tasting, as they are medicinal and potent. Just because an herb tastes unpleasant to you does not necessarily mean it is a poor choice for you.

5

The Food-Mood Relationship to Organ Dysfunction

Last but not least important, there is another way to look at illness and the imbalances it causes. This can be another clue in determining the cause of your illness. In Chinese medicine, the organs when out of balance correspond to certain emotions, as well as physical symptoms. While common, daily changes in moods are normal, extremes in emotions are not, nor are exaggerated responses to everyday situations. Pent-up emotions can be caused by a disharmonious energy in the body's organs. This is also true in Ayurvedic medicine. In relationship to natural healing, food turns into energy that affects the organs and then the emotions. Foods, as we learned, contain certain energetic properties. Everything is a form of energy in one way or another. In its slow state, water is basically visible energy to the naked eye. It its fast state, boiling water changes to steam which makes it an almost invisible form of energy. These symptoms of organ disharmony can give you insight into part of the cause of your medical problem.

The Liver/Gall bladder– When its energy is in disharmony or stagnation, a person will have a tendency to get irritated, angry, and agitated easily. Often "lashing out" is common, or anger is exaggerated and unjustifiable. Breast soreness, right before the menstrual period and irregular menstrual cycles are other symptoms of stagnant liver qi, along with shoulder and neck muscle tension, and possible tenderness below the rib cage over the liver area (your right side of the body). Chronic headaches and migraines are another sign of liver trouble (traditionally called liver yang rising), along with the obvious medical disorders such as jaundice, hepatitis, elevated liver enzymes, high cholesterol, and gallstones. A visible sign of liver disharmony on the face is having deep longitudinal lines/vertical wrinkles between the eyebrows. In cases where the liver begins to affect digestion (a condition called liver invading the spleen), gas and bloating may be present.

Foods that aggravate the liver are spicy, sour, and fermented. Basically, pitta increasing foods are aggravating to the liver. Bitter leafy greens like plenty of salads, kale, dandelion, parsley, spinach, lettuce, collards, and broccoli, sprouts, okra, artichokes, asparagus, avocado, and olive oil actually help this organ. Raw foods are great for the liver too. Pitta reducing type foods nicely release a stagnated liver. Bitter herbs such as milk thistle, golden seal, turmeric, echinacea, burdock root, bhumy amalaki, neem, gentian root, aloe vera gel, chicory, lemon balm, chrysanthemum, peppermint, and bupleurum help this organ function smoothly.

The Lungs/Large Intestine – When the lungs are aggravated with water and mucus buildup, and there also may be mucus in the stools, watery or greasy stools. The person will often feel lethargic, depressed or sad. Crying streaks are common, as well as the inability to think clearly. Breathing in humid weather will be difficult. Foods that aggravate this condition are: too much damp mucus producing foods such as dairy products, rice, oatmeal, winter squashes, zucchini, cucumbers, melons, bananas, sour foods like lemons, yogurt, tomatoes; oily foods like cheeses, nuts and sweet heavy pastries and desserts; and too much liquid. Pungent and spicy foods help this problem like daikon and red radishes, onions, leeks, chives, garlic, ginger, turnips, kohlrabi, mushrooms, burdock, as well as more drying grains like buckwheat, corn, barley, millet, and rye bread. Pungent and drying herbs for this type of damp lung disorder are: garlic, ginger, sage, elecampane, bayberry bark, mullein, red raspberry leaf, eucalyptus, pippali, trikatu, cayenne, vasaka, shilajit, cinnamon, clove, punarnava, cleavers, black pepper, and fenugreek.

Sometimes the lung tissues can become aggravated and damaged by too many dry foods and beverages. This type of lung disorder is an opposite condition compared to the one just described above, and is more common in vata individuals whose bodies physically tend towards dryness. Sensitivity to smoke, incense, ragweed, dust particles, or a wood burning stove can be clues. In the large intestine and colon, bloating, gas, and chronic constipation may also be present. In this case, just the opposite recommendations will apply such as emphasizing moistening substances: fruit juices, pineapple, orange, grape, pear, coconut, lemon, and lime. Rice, oatmeal, wheat, and dairy products will help lubricate dry airway passages making breathing easier. Moist vegetables like zucchini, winter squashes, tomato sauce, yams, cucumbers, and artichokes help, along with nuts. Herbs that restore moisture to the lungs and large intestine are: licorice root, marshmallow, Solomon's seal, shatavari, bala, kapikacchu, slippery elm, rehmannia, codonopsis, vamsha rochana, amalaki, and comfrey tea.

The Heart/Small intestine - A person with an imbalance here is likely to feel too much joy (they get excited too easily), have hyperactivity, insomnia, may be very boisterous, have heart palpitations, heart trouble, possible chest pains, circulatory problems, blood pressure problems, and sometimes, but not always, a bulbous swollen purple nose. When a person has lost that sense of spirit, vitality in their eyes, and they have anxiety, think too much, are overly sensitive to their environment, the person has a disturbed "shen" or spirit in relationship to the heart, according to Chinese medicine. Generally, substances that aggravate the heart are elevated cholesterol and triglyceride levels. However, there are some other factors that play a role depending on the person (body type).

In vata type individuals, hyperactivity, palpitations, and insomnia are often common. Vata types suffer from insomnia more than any other body type. The vata women often experience blood deficiency as well, which can affect the heart causing insomnia right before the menstrual period. Signs of blood deficiency affecting the heart are: a pale face, scanty menses, dry hair and skin, a weak pulse, possible dizziness, especially upon standing, along with insomnia, heart palpitations, and anxiety. Too many bitters and astringent foods aggravate the heart in these people, disturbing its energy and shen. Foods which benefit this condition are slightly sour such as oranges, pineapple, green grapes, plums, cherries, mangoes, bananas, lemons, limes, peaches, tomatoes, kiwis, yogurt. Aside from consuming more sour type foods, the vata person can take hawthorn berries to strengthen the heart muscle. Sweet foods also have a calming action, as well as nourishing action in these types of people. Both sweet and sour foods and herbs counteract the vata tendency towards blood deficiency and disturbed shen affecting the heart. Garlic and a few other pungent herbs and spices can help improve circulation and blood flow. Heavier herbs that sedate heart palpitations in the case of a disturbed "shen" and help reverse insomnia are biota seeds, shatavari, ashwagandha, licorice root, marshmallow, Solomon's seal, hawthorn berries, codonopsis, jatamansi, and zizyphus. Over work and too much exercise or exertion should be avoided.

Pitta people tend to have different signs of heart trouble such as signs of heat and possible dryness or what the Chinese call "yin deficiency." Symptoms, such as a red face, high blood pressure, extreme thirst, a red tongue, night sweats, irritability and anger if the liver is involved, will be present. There may also be insomnia, nightmares, and restlessness involved. (In vata people, heat related health problems are not as common, but they too, can have this problem.) In the pitta type case above, sweet, bitter and cooling foods will actually help, such as plenty of leafy greens, milk, ice cream, wheat products, winter squashes, sweet fruits such as apples, dates, pears, and purple grapes. Too much garlic and hot spices should be avoided, as well as fermented and sour foods. Pitta people should cut back on their meat consumption, as meat generates heat in the body. Bitter herbs such as aloe vera, brahmi, bhumy amalaki, dandelion, golden seal, and neem cool heated emotions, heated blood, and lower blood pressure and high cholesterol. Sweet cool herbs that calm the shen, counteract dryness caused from too much heat drying up fluids, are: shatavari, licorice root, Solomon's seal, vamsha rochana, the Western herb wild yam, and slippery elm. Arjuna is a better choice for strengthening the heart muscle, as it is not sour like hawthorn berries.

Kapha people seem most affected by fatty diets and hence, a low fat diet is recommended. Pastries, fatty desserts, fatty dairy products and meats should be cut back or avoided. Bitter and pungent herbs that break down fats, weight, and water, will benefit them (dandelion, golden seal, gentian, garlic, ginger, cayenne, aloe vera, bhumy amalaki, neem, pippali, punarnava, uva ursi, and guggul). Arjuna can be taken for heart strength. Exercise is extremely beneficial for these type of people. Check with your physician first to okay it if you suspect a problem.

The Stomach/Pancreas/Spleen – Diabetes and hypoglycemia (blood sugar dysfunctions) are diseases related to a malfunctioning pancreas. Signs of a disturbed stomach and spleen are bloating and or gas after eating, nausea, loss of appetite, diarrhea, constipation, or excessive appetite and thirst. Foods and herbs that help strengthen these organs are different, depending on one's body type, and medical condition. Below are just some general suggestions. However, to effectively treat these organs, you must first identify the specific condition: diarrhea, constipation, gas/bloating, nausea or too much acidity.

For diabetes, the herb licorice root benefits vata and pitta people, and most diabetics will benefit from the use of bitter herbs such as neem, gentian, dandelion, golden seal, and gurmar, as they help pancreatic function. Also what is fascinating to me, is that pitta people in general, have a much higher biological need for naturally sweet foods, than others, in order to sustain normal blood sugar levels, while kapha predominant people are the most biologically susceptible to developing diabetes and have the least physical tolerance for naturally sweet foods - although anyone can develop diabetes. Kapha type people seem to have greater insulin sensitivity. Glucose sensitivity and insulin response is different in people depending on their body type. (In my own personal case, being predominantly pitta, this is true. Years ago, I watched my body's blood sugar return to normal after adding back in white sugar, sweet fruit juices, sweet fruits such as dates, red apples, red grapes, cherries, pears, soda, ice cream and other desserts with white sugar. The omission of these foods in my diet for several years had caused me to be extremely hypoglycemic at one point in my life).

In vata people, herbs that generally treat gas, bloating and constipation are: cumin, salt, lemon, lime, asafoetida, ginger, black pepper, cinnamon, cardamom, haritaki, fennel, licorice root, triphala, amalaki, castor oil, marshmallow, and Solomon's seal. The latter seven herbs are laxative/moisture restoring, while the first ten herbs act as carminatives (dispel gas). Again, foods and herbs that are spicy, salty, sour and sweet help most vata digestive problems, including a little yogurt with lunch or wine with dinner as they are sour and fermented.

In pitta people, too much acidity is often a common digestive complaint, along with loose stools or dry stools. Cumin, fennel, and coriander can help dispel gas from fermentation and too much acidity in the digestive tract. Many natural anti-acids are available such as slippery elm, licorice, shatavari, neem, turmeric, red clover, peppermint, chamomile, etc. For loose stools, the diet needs to be drier and void of spicy, sour or fermented foods. Bitter and astringent herbs will help bind up the stools such as red raspberry leaf, agrimony, chamomile, mullein, ashoka, neem, and musta. For hard stools, use slippery elm, licorice, marshmallow, or shatavari. If the liver is involved (look for yellow stools), then more liver regulating herbs and foods are needed such as turmeric, aloe, bhumy amalaki, neem, gentian, golden seal, burdock, dandelion, chlorophyll.

Generally speaking, in kapha people, too many processed, refined sugars, along with too many naturally sweet foods, will weaken the pancreas. Kapha types are also most susceptible to what the Chinese call dampness in the spleen/stomach. Since their bodies tend to naturally produce more oil, mucus, and water, a diet containing too many wet, heavy, sweet and greasy foods will set them up for loose stools, or nausea. Other symptoms of dampness in the gut are: a greasy thick coating on the tongue, mucus in the stools, and water retention. Edema (swelling) in the fingers/hands, although normal after exercise and in hot weather, is often a disturbance of the spleen. The spleen, along with the kidneys, is responsible for water metabolism in the body. To disrupt its function is to disrupt the transport and circulation of water, especially in the central part of the body, like the hands.

A reduction of sweet, oily, and sour foods in the diet will help immensely such as avoiding (sugar, dairy products, winter squashes, yams/sweet potatoes, pumpkin, tomatoes/sauce, cucumbers, zucchini, avocado, bananas, lemons, limes, grapefruit, kiwis, oranges, pineapple, melons, coconut, dates, figs, mangoes, oatmeal, cream of wheat, tofu/soy products, and sweet fruit juices). Herbs for the kapha stomach/pancreas/spleen, are: pungent herbs such as ginger, basil, trikatu, pippali, atractylodes, saussurea, aurantium, magnolia, and bitters such as dandelion, bupleurum, turmeric, neem, punarnava, bhumy amalaki, or aloe vera. Even diuretics such as dandelion, uva ursi, cornsilk, juniper berries, cranberry, shilajit, parsley, and cleavers are helpful. Many good Chinese herbal diuretic formulas are now on the market. The herbs above are all drying in general, and break up mucus and mass, hence they are great for nausea. A few days of eating lighter foods or fasting will help the gut tremendously.

The Kidneys/Bladder – Fear is the emotion associated with unbalanced energy in the kidneys. This organ has several patterns of disharmony that can manifest from it. The Chinese consider the kidneys as the "life gate," the foundation of the entire body and its functions. General kidney deficiency symptoms are: chronic dizziness, ringing in the ears, loss of sexual libido, general fatigue, hair loss, sore weak lower back, and weak knees. Another pattern, called kidney yin deficiency, has symptoms of heat such as thirst, red face, dark scanty urine possible urinary tract infections; along with dry symptoms: constipation, dry throat/mouth, dry hair, etc. Possible general kidney deficiency signs listed above, may occur simultaneously with kidney yin deficiency. Symptoms of kidney yang deficiency (a cold condition affecting the kidneys) are: cold hands and feet, lack of thirst, pale tongue, pale skin, edema, frequent urination, nighttime urination, urine dribbling, and sometimes back pain over the kidney region. Kidney yang deficiency may or may not be accompanied by general kidney deficiency. When this type of yang deficiency disorder is present, exposure to cold weather, cold temperature foods and drinks, cooling herbs, and foods should be avoided. The area on the body associated with the kidneys is the area around the eyes on the face. When this area becomes darkened, this is usually a sign of kidney disharmony. Puffiness under the eyes indicates a different type of disharmony of the kidneys from the drinking of too many fluids.

Too many, as well as too little liquids can be detrimental to the kidneys. Warm cooked foods, warming spices, and foods that have a warming energy effect on the body strengthen the kidneys from cold. See the advice in this book for foods for cold hands and feet, and urinary frequency. Salty foods are also good for cold overactive kidneys, but not when there is edema. General herbs which benefit the kidney and bladder in a case of extreme coldness in that region (kidney yang deficiency) are: saw palmetto, Chinese ginseng, ashwagandha, cistanche stem, cooked rehmannia root, cynomorium stem, fenugreek seed, teasel root, shilajit, eucommia bark, garlic, cinnamon bark, ginger root, walnut, psoralea fruit, cuscuta seed, dipsacus root, and morinda root, just to mention a few. For kidney yin deficiency, cooling herbs will help such as: shatavari root, ophiopogon root, fo-ti, marshmallow root, raw rehmannia root, lycium fruit, Solomon's seal, uva ursi, cleavers, dandelion, cornsilk. Cleavers and uva ursi are drying/diuretic and should not be used in dry heat cases but in cases of damp heat in the bladder/kidney region. Often vata, and vata-pitta types will have symptoms of either kidney yin or yang deficiency sin which case, Chinese formulas such as rehmannia 8 for kidney yang deficiency and rehmannia 6 for kidney yin deficiency, will be helpful. These type of formulas warm and moisten at the same time, or cool and moisten.

6

59 Common Medical Problems, Their Causes, and Suggested Treatments (An A-Z List)

1) Acne

Cause: This imbalance in the system is usually caused from excess Pitta. Oily, fatty foods aggravate it as well as too many sour and fermented foods and foods that feed inflammation, bacteria, and infection in the skin. High pitta is almost synonymous with infection. It is important to remember that to treat acne effectively, you must treat it from the inside out, at the blood level, not topically/externally only.

Treatment: Emphasize more bitter, astringent, and naturally sweet foods like kale, collards, lettuce, spinach, sprouts, peas, broccoli, green beans, asparagus, zucchini, cabbage, cauliflower, white potatoes, red apples, pears, purple grapes, plums, cherries, dates, figs, honeydew, watermelon, beans, skim milk, vanilla ice cream, nonfat cottage cheese (mainly more pitta reducing foods). Avoid greasy, oily, fatty foods such as French fries, fried foods, peanut butter, nuts, potato chips, baked goods with lots of fat, etc. Switch from whole milk to skim, etc. Also try herbs that are blood cleansers and stop infection such as red clover, dandelion, neem, golden seal, bhumy amalaki, gentian root, or aloe vera gel, for 1-3 months. Aloe vera gel can be taken internally and used externally. It is an excellent natural blood and skin cleanser. You can try ¼ cup a day internally for a few weeks, and also apply it topically to the infected areas on your skin. For acne with oily skin, also try applying rubbing alcohol to the skin. If you are vata predominant, consider taking some heavier tonic herbs, to keep your balance, while using the above blood cleansers. Herbal formulas for the vata person can consist of bala, shatavari, marshmallow, or licorice along with neem, red clover, or golden seal.

2) Allergies (food and environmental)

Cause: Allergies are caused by a weak immune system, but the key to strengthening your immune system is to strengthen your body type/constitution, and correct the underlying imbalance. So in this case, just simply taking anti-oxidants and immune boosting supplements will not work. Everybody has a different physiological makeup and specific and unique nutritional needs to keep it in balance. The more in balance an individual is, the less likely they will have allergies. Often times, individuals will react to substances such as particular foods or environmental conditions that are wrong for their unique biological system to begin with, and the more out of balance they are, the more strongly they will react to those substances. Two examples of this are people with excessive internal dryness like vata people who begin reacting allergically to dust or smoke, or a child with a cold, damp kapha type of asthma who experiences attacks during cold/damp rainy seasons. Hence, cold damp foods will aggravate the latter condition. The more internally damp the kid, the more likely the asthma will flare up. Recovery for this child then will depend on a dryer diet, and plenty of warm dry heat.

The same thing for food allergies. Allergies to fermented foods can occur when an individual is naturally internally sour/acidic to begin with, such as a pitta predominant person. When out of balance, this person will have a tendency to be more acidic and hence be more sensitive to fermented foods, because those foods are naturally sour. The pitta predominant individual usually cannot digest fermented foods well to begin with, without bloating/gas. Therefore, sour foods and fermented substances stagnant in the digestive tract causing allergic reactions.

The key to recovery here, is to strengthen your body type by reducing its excess tendencies internally. If you naturally have a tendency to be dry internally and externally on your skin, balance your system by restoring internal moisture, and your allergy to dry airborne particles such as smoke, incense, or dry heat/wind will disappear or lessen. If you have a physically tendency to be internally damp, such as the kapha predominant person, then by literally drying yourself up internally will help diminish your hay fever, allergies, or asthma.

Treatment: Follow the appropriate diet and lifestyle program for your own body and/or physical imbalance. Vata people or people with a vata imbalance such as too much dryness in their system should be on vata reducing foods and lifestyle plans to strengthen their immune system. Pitta people or people with pitta imbalances should avoid things that increase pitta, and so on.

Generally, because vata people usually develop allergies to ragweed, dust, or smoke that are dry airborne particles, restoring internal moisture as well as taking immune boosters specifically for vata will help. Licorice root, ashwagandha, amalaki, kapikacchu, rehmannia, bala, codonopsis, shatavari, fo-ti, Solomon's seal, marshmallow, are all good herbs for doing both. Look for herbal formulas that are made up mostly of these types of herbs. In Chinese medicine, these herbs are called qi tonics, meaning they boost strength, vitality, energy, and immunity. In Ayurveda, they simply reduce vata, and by doing so, do the same thing. Avoid dry type of foods. Vitamins: Beta

Carotene, C, D, and E as well as minerals, help strengthen vata, as well as eating more moistening, heavy, warm cooked foods like those in the vata diet.

Pitta people should avoid sour and fermented foods such as strawberries, papaya, kiwi, lemons, limes, tangerines, grapefruit, pickles, yogurt, coffee, alcohol, tempeh, soy sauce, miso, sourdough breads. Vitamin C is the one vitamin that pittas do not benefit much from because of its acidity. The diet should contain plenty of naturally sweet foods and salads. They can also strengthen their immune system in other ways by taking herbal formulas with much shatavari, licorice root, Solomon's seal, fo-ti, kapikacchu, bala, wild yam, and/or rehmannia root. These herbs will help give them strength when there is weakness in the body, as well as restore moisture when there is dryness. If infection, heat, or inflammation are present, the temporarily use of bitters will help clear them, such as aloe vera, dandelion, neem, golden seal, yellow dock, red clover, gentian root, echinacea, and bhumy amalaki. Do not use these bitters for prolonged periods of time. The B vitamins help decrease inflammation in the body and can sometimes be beneficial.

Kapha people should be on kapha reducing foods and lifestyle programs. Often they do not need super heavy vitamin and mineral supplementation because they have the tendency to suffer from health problems related to excess. Their immune system can benefit from bitter herbs used occasionally such as dandelion, turmeric, guduchi, aloe vera, echinacea, golden seal, burdock, red clover, neem, and spicy pungent herbs like garlic, ginger, clove, cinnamon, cayenne, pippali, black pepper. In general, the bitter herbs will help with inflammation, infection, dry up secretions, help break down fats, while the pungent spicy herbs will help break up stagnation, mucus, improve circulation. The temporarily use of diuretics can help decrease dampness in the respiratory tract, thus helping damp types of asthma or sinus problems. These include: uva ursi, dandelion, cornsilk, cleavers, shilajit, juniper berries, and parsley. Vasaka, sage, bayberry, wild cherry bark, mullein, eucalyptus, peppermint, and basil are good herbs for drying up wet congested lungs and sinuses.

3) Anemia

Cause: There are several causes for this condition as well as pitta and vata specific types of anemia. In vata type anemia, the person usually has a deficient condition whereas they don't produce enough blood as well as having qi deficiency (lack of energy, stamina, strength, vitality). Dizziness, scanty menstrual flow, a pale complexion, a thready weak pulse, a pale tongue, are some other signs of deficient blood. The tongue could be flabby in qi deficiency cases. Sometimes the person will also have dry skin, numbness in the fingers and palpitations or insomnia. Vata types are most prone to this disorder as they tend to develop deficiency related diseases.

In pitta or pitta-kapha type anemia, the person may have anemia due to excessive bleeding since that is their biological tendency. Cases like these are often caused from a type of hemorrhaging - usually blood leaking from vessels or veins in the body. Excess heat is often the culprit, as heat causes blood to move quicker and leak. However, pitta type people can also have a vata type anemia, if they have a temporary vata imbalance. In anemia, due to bleeding, one must stop the bleeding to reverse this problem.

Treatment: For the vata type anemia - foods high in iron, as well as following a heavy nourishing, moistening, and tonifying vata reducing diet will help. Malnourishment is usually the cause for this problem. Blood building foods are: beets, yams, black strap molasses, black/red/purple grapes/juice, bananas, melons, kiwis, lemonade, peaches, plums, oranges, pineapple, mangoes, dates, nuts, oatmeal, seaweeds, beef, organ meats, seafood, oatmeal, brown rice, wheat products, winter squashes, tomatoes, zucchini, avocado, cucumbers, spinach, yogurt, milk, cottage cheese, ice cream. Iron supplements, or Indian herb formulas like chywan prash are good. Liver tablets are also helpful. Herbs to help build both blood and qi in the body are: fo-ti, rehmannia root, shatavari, marshmallow, lycium fruit, licorice, codonopsis, jujube fruit, mulberry fruit, longan fruit, and wild yam. Some herbs to help circulate the blood, as well as add warmth when there is physical coldness present are: angelica, paeonia root, milletia root, ligusticum, ginger, cinnamon, cardamom, garlic, pennyroyal. Warm qi tonics such as Chinese ginseng, ashwagandha, and astragalus can also be added. Again, the cause of this is deficiency, so to reverse this, the diet must be highly nutritive and nutritiously dense such as a vata diet.

For pitta type anemia: Use hemostatics (herbs that stop bleeding) and cooling herbs such as manjistha, red raspberry leaf, plantain, agrimony, musta, or ashoka. Basically, any herb that is astringent, bitter, drying, and cooling can help stop bleeding, including dandelion and neem. Yellow dock is an herb that has iron in it naturally, and also stops bleeding. Be cautious. Do not overdose on iron. Too much iron is toxic and thought to accelerate cancer. Stick with the RDA recommended amount such as 18 mg if you are considering a supplement. Be sure to also follow more of a pitta reducing diet (a diet emphasizing these foods will naturally contain many astringent and bitter foods as well as foods that are more cooling). Avoid hot spicy spices as these heat up the blood. Also avoid sour and heavy foods, since these types of foods will make the menstrual blood flow volume heavier, such as too many grapefruits, lemons, limes, kiwis, bananas, pineapple, oranges, papaya, yogurt, sour cream, cottage cheese, pickles, alcohol, tomatoes, winter squashes, yams/sweet potatoes, zucchini, and avocado.

4) Anxiety

Cause: True anxiety is long term and chronic, which can cause heart palpitations, hyperventilating, over-excitability, some weight loss, possible tremors, numbness or tingling in the hands, butterfly stomach feeling, abnormal phobias about everyday normal stress or situations, etc. This condition can be caused from psychological issues or a physical chemical imbalance such as high vata in the system, deficient nerve tissue. It requires strong nourishment to the body. In Chinese medicine it is seen as a disturbance of the heart or "shen." Anxiety is often the opposite medical condition of some types, but not all kinds of depression in which the person is not grounded enough and feels "hyperactive," or has too much nervous energy, and insomnia. Pitta and kapha people can experience anxiety, although it is more unlikely in kapha types, and almost always purely psychological.

Treatment: **For the vata type described above**: Avoiding traveling and too much aerobic exercise. Try aromatherapy treatments with calming fragrances such as vanilla, lavender, frankincense, and sandalwood. Massage therapy is also beneficial. Listen to calming music such as nature sound tapes and CDs. Follow a daily routine to ground oneself. In your surroundings put objects around you that make you feel safe. Sleep with a heavy blanket covering you. This helps ground you.

Eat heavier foods to nourish yourself such as vata reducing foods. Temporarily avoid too many salads, leafy greens, beans/legumes, cornbread, corn chips, popcorn, pretzels, crackers, granola, rye bread, millet, amaranth, quinoa, radishes, turnips, broccoli, cauliflower, cabbage, kale, cranberries/juice, and most herbal teas. Emphasize rice, wheat, and cooked oats, dairy products such as cottage cheese, yogurt, milk, tofu, eggs, winter squashes, tomatoes, zucchini, summer squash, cucumbers, pumpkin, spaghetti squash, artichokes, kiwis, lemonade, bananas, grapes, plums, fresh apricots, peaches, melons, coconut , red apples, pears, dates, figs, mangoes, bananas, plantains, nuts, chocolate, sweet foods/desserts, and plenty of sweet juices. One word of warning: too much heavy food for long periods of time can cause nausea and a diminished appetite. If this starts to happen, balance out with some lighter foods again. Also take tonic heavy herbs to build up and nourish the nervous tissue such as: up like shatavari, ashwagandha, kapikacchu, hawthorn berries, wild yam, ginseng, marshmallow, codonopsis root, cotton root, jujube, Solomon's seal, kapikacchu, licorice, slippery elm, fo-ti, 2 capsules 2-3 times a day. Since these heavy herbs tend to be congesting, you might want to try a combination of these herbs with a little ginger, cinnamon, orange peel, or cardamom added, or look for a formula with a similar makeup. The herb zizyphus is a strong, sweet, sour vata nerve tonic and sedative as well. You may want to try 1 capsule or tablet 3 times a day for a month or so. If you have insomnia, try valerian, 1-2 capsules with warm milk and nutmeg at bedtime, or 1/4 –3/4 tsp. jatamansi before bed (both of these herbs are sedatives). Jatamansi is better for pitta types. Exercise caution when taking them, and never operate a car under their influence. Simply drinking 1 cup of warm milk with 1/4 teaspoon of nutmeg, 2 T of poppy seeds and 1 teaspoon of white sugar might do the trick for mild insomnia. If still having trouble sleeping, take a warm bath for 20 minutes in the evening regularly. If you have low blood pressure, exercise caution: the warm water can make you dizzy and lower blood pressure.

Also, do not label yourself as an individual with an anxiety condition. This only keeps you focused on your medical condition and can scare you into a hyperventilation attack. It feeds a vicious cycle. Learn to see yourself as a normal individual who is legitimately reacting to some of life's stressors. Do not pay attention to the increase in your heart rate. This can also cause fear, and feed the cycle, by causing you to breath faster and then start to hyperventilate. One method to break this cycle, is to pick a mantra (a word or phrase to repeat), that has a feeling or meaning of safety and courage for you. Repeat the mantra during the cycle. Another method is to visualize a serene, peaceful, safe place, whether it be walking on the ocean beach or sitting in a meadow or forest. Use whatever works for you. Take deep breaths and use a paper bag to breathe into if you must to slow your breathing down. The carbon dioxide will help you slow your breathing down. Remember, these suggestions are only coping skills. To reverse true anxiety, you must treat the root cause by building and strengthening the nervous system, and/or treating any underlying psychological issue, perhaps through counseling.

For pitta type anxiety: Try using some of the heavy nerve tonics such as rehmannia, shatavari, licorice root, bala, red date, codonopsis root, or ho-shou-wu in a formula with other herbs. You may also try jatamansi at bedtime as a sedative in doses of 1/4 to 3/4 tsp. Again, exercise caution, as this herb acts like an opiate. Do not take it with any sedatives, alcohol, or while driving a car.

Kapha type anxiety: Try kava kava, or jatamansi at bedtime (1-2 capsules). Kava kava is a strong sedative used for anxiety. Do not take any other sleeping pills, sedatives

or pain killers with it, and exercise caution. Do not operate a car under its influence.
A tea made from skullcap, catnip, hops and thyme can be taken to calm and mildly sedate the nerves. St. John's Wort during the day, could be an added measure.

5) Arthritis

Cause: There are many different types of arthritis and causes for each of them. To effectively treat your arthritis, look to the specific symptoms and specific type of pain or discomfort. For example, do your joints crack and pop and is the pain very sharp, or burning? Is there a dull constant pain that improves with exercise but feels worse when you first get out of bed? Does damp hot weather make your condition worse? Is there stiffness associated with your joints and muscles? Is there any swelling or distinctive redness on your skin? Do sour, acid, and spicy foods like cranberry juice, chilies, tomatoes, oranges and coffee make the pain worse?

Generally, most pain associated with arthritis, is caused from inflammation or excess heat in the joints and muscles. Inflammation can be present with either rheumatoid arthritis or osteoarthritis. Kapha types tend to get swelling or edema with inflammation pain, vata types tend to get cartilage deterioration with inflammation, and pitta types can get either. Most importantly, the greater the inflammation or heat, the stronger or sharper the pain. All heat caused from excess pitta in the body.

Treatment: For kapha type arthritis with stiffness, a dull aching pain, and swelling around the joints that also improves with exercise and activity, follow a kapha/pitta related diet, avoiding foods and substances that cause dampness, mucus, fat, heat, and congestion to build up in the system. These types of foods can cause stagnation, heat, and blockages in the system, leading to that dull, heavy, aching, sore feeling. Use diuretics, as well as bitters. Cooling diuretics include: uva ursi, dandelion, cleavers, cornsilk, or punarnava. Bitter herbs that decrease inflammation include: golden seal, neem, bhumy amalaki, gentian root, or aloe vera. Sour cream yogurt, cheese, citrus fruits, bananas, tomatoes, coffee, alcohol, and hot spices strongly aggravate this type of arthritis, and should be avoided. For temporary natural pain relief, try 1-2 capsules of white willow bark provided you are not allergic to aspirin. If allergic to aspirin, try a tea brewed from 1 teaspoon of the following herbs: skullcap, catnip, hops and peppermint (1-2 cups a day). These herbs are all mild nerve sedatives and reduce heat. In theory, cold ice packs applied externally help inflammatory pain. Oddly, some people report that heat applications help, such as hot ginger compresses or pastes made from camphor, menthol, wintergreen, ginger, eucalyptus, or pine. If using essential oils, mix them with some vegetable oil. In my experience, a simple paste of dry ginger root and water spread over the dull aching area and left on for 15 minutes, is an excellent temporary and inexpensive remedy. For a stronger plaster you can mix dry mustard powder with wheat flour, making sure to include enough flour since too much mustard can burn the skin. Tiger balm is an excellent topical choice as well!

For pitta people, with severe burning, inflammatory type pain, and/or redness, avoid sour, heating, and fermented foods along with spicy foods. These will cause a flare up in any type of inflammation. Emphasize a pitta type diet that will cool down heat and inflammation. Try cooling herbs such as: neem, golden seal, gentian root, bhumy amalaki, aloe, mints, or dandelion, with heavier cooling herbs such as: shatavari, marshmallow, licorice, bala, or fo-ti. The first seven herbs are much more cooling and put out inflammation more aggressively. Many excellent Chinese herbal formulas also exist for inflammatory type pain and are appropriately named "purge fire" or "clear heat." Exercise caution and do not use bitter herbs while also on blood thinning medication or if taking vitamin E in large doses. White willow bark can also be taken specifically as a pain reliever, or tea brewed from skullcap, catnip, and peppermint. The Indian herb jatamansi is a nerve sedative that can be used for inflammatory pain. (Never use valerian, as it increases heat.) Externally apply ice to the site of pain or bathe in cool water. To help stop or slow any bone loss due to too much acidity, try calcium magnesium supplements with vitamin D. You might also want to try glucosamine sulfate and chrondroitin for osteoarthritis.

For cracking or deterioration of the joints, stiffness, and inflammatory pain, follow more of a vata or vata/pitta reducing diet. Try bone and joint building type herbs such as: marshmallow, shatavari, bala, licorice, Solomon's seal, or fo-ti. Try 2 capsules 3 times a day. As said before, vata type arthritis tends to be degenerative. The herb amalaki and vitamin C should be added to help improve flexibility in the joints and muscle tissues, as well as slow cartilage breakdown. Cold herbs will reverse inflammation such as golden seal, neem or gentian root. The diet should contain extra vegetable oil or nuts. Evening primrose oil is good as a supplement. Glucosamine sulfate and chrondroitin might help slow cartilage loss. Self massage the skin with coconut oil. In vata types of arthritis, warm, moist heat will make it feel better, or try a ginger compress or ginger and water paste over the area externally. To do this bring a large pot of water to almost a boil. Grate a grapefruit size ball of ginger root and tie with a rubber band in a cheesecloth. Squeeze the ginger juice into the hot water, then let the whole ball drop into the pot. Turn the heat off. When hot, but not scalding, dip a small towel or dish rag into the ginger bath, holding it by both ends and letting the center dip into the bath. Wring out some of the extra water. Apply directly to the area, covering with another towel to hold in the heat. Repeat the procedure when the towel touching the skin becomes cool. Try this for 20 minutes. The heat helps the pain, while the ginger will improve the circulation in that area. To make a simple ginger paste, simply mix dry ginger root and warm water, then apply directly over the are, leaving on for 15 minutes. Tiger balm is a great topical treatment for pain. Hot tubs are also excellent as are plain hot water baths in which most of the body is submerged. Good supplements for this condition are vitamins A, C, D, E, plus a calcium/magnesium formula. Consume plenty of dairy products like ice cream and milk, nuts, winter squashes, yams, zucchini, cucumbers, avocado, oatmeal, white rice, wheat breads, sweet fruits, and juices.

6) Asthma

Cause: There are many different causes for this serious medical condition and many different types of asthma. The cause and treatment depend on which type you have. There are dry vata types with no mucus and dry wheezing, damp types with heat or infection present, such as thick to watery sputum with yellow, green, or blood streaks, and cold damp types which have thick white mucus. The damp types will be aggravated in humidity or on rainy days. The dry types will be most agitated in the fall or dry season. Dry climates, like that of deserts, will aggravate dry asthma. On average, vata people tend to have dry types of asthma, pitta people tend toward either damp heat or dry heat types, and kapha people usually have damp, thick, white phlegm types. Kapha/pitta people will usually have damp heat types.

Treatment: For vata dry type asthma, follow a vata reducing diet. Try herbs that are lubricating and moistening to the lungs such as: vamsha rochana, bala, kapikacchu, marshmallow, Solomon's seal, wild yam, slippery elm, shatavari, and licorice root. Try 1/2-3/4 teaspoon three times a day or 2-3 capsules three times a day. Vitamin C, the herb amalaki, and hawthorn berries are sour herbs that will also alleviate internal dryness and strengthen lung tissue. Fennel powder is both a spice and moistening herb that can be made into a tea or taken in capsule form. Moistening drinks such as grapefruit juice, lemonade, orange juice, pineapple, coconut, or purple grape juice are great. Avoid the sour juices if you have an ulcer or chronic heartburn. Herbs that are bronchidilators can help open airway passages. They are: eucalyptus, peppermint, and ephedra. Eucalyptus and peppermint are much safer to use than ephedra, which can cause heart palpitations, anxiety, nervousness, insomnia, and high blood pressure. (Ephedra should never be used by people with those disorders, heart problems, or hypertension. It should be used only under the supervision and care of a practitioner or physician.) Although ephedra is one of the strongest brochidilators available, sadly there has been several reported deaths from its use. If you do decide to use it, exercise extreme caution and use it in small doses. It is a very strong stimulant. There are also natural herbal inhalers available on the market, although I personally believe they are too weak. Regular bathing in plain bathtub water or a lake or pond can help you rehydrate. Especially avoid dry foods like corn chips, pretzels, broccoli, cauliflower, cabbage, Brussels sprouts, beans, peas, too many raw apples, berries. All of your foods should be somewhat soft, moist, and juicy!

For the pitta type of asthma: If your cough tends to be dry, hacking, or hoarse without much mucus, use moistening cooling lung herbs such as equal amounts of vamsha rochana and bala, or licorice, codonopsis root, kapikacchu, Solomon's seal, marshmallow, shatavari and bala. Try 1/2 teaspoon three times a day with honey as a paste or 2 capsules three times a day. Try a tea made from equal parts eucalyptus, licorice and mint to help open breathing passages. Fennel capsules can also be used as they are moistening. For a heavier, damp type of asthma in the pitta person, who has thick white sputum or mucus, try more drying herbs such as a tea or capsules made from mullein leaf and peppermint. Include 1/4 teaspoon vasaka powder or 1 capsule three times a day to decongest the sinuses and lungs. If there is internal infection evident by green, or yellow coloring in the mucus, try bitter herbal antibiotics for three weeks or until the infection disappears. Such herbs are: golden seal, neem, echinacea, or bhumy amalaki. Dosages can consist of 1 capsule taken three to four times a day, depending on body weight.

Kapha types of asthma need drying and circulatory promoting foods and substances. Herbally, try 1-3 cups of tea a day of equal parts mullein, thyme, sage, eucalyptus, mint, and elecampane, or bayberry, cloves, horehound, cornsilk, and mullein. (Brew 1 teaspoon of herbs per cup of water. Strain, sweeten with honey, and drink.) Ephedra is a strong brochidilator for the lungs, and can be added to your cup of tea such as a pinch of the dried herb. However, as I said above, it is one of the strongest stimulating herbs available and one needs to exercise caution when using it. Again, avoid it if you have a history of heart problems, hypertension, irregular heartbeat, anxiety, or insomnia. Also try equal parts of vasaka and trikatu, vasaka and pippali, or vasaka and ginger (1/4 teaspoon three times a day). A blend of turmeric, clove, ginger and black pepper with honey, will also help break up mucus. Other suggestions include Chinese lotus root tea, as it is very drying. Pour 1 cup of hot water over 1 teaspoon of the powdered lotus root, and drink 1 cup a day. Spicy teas, coffee, and/or grain chicory coffee substitutes are excellent in the diet, along with horseradish. For starters, strictly avoid dairy products, citrus, tomatoes, and bananas. These aggravate heavy mucus production. Be sure to also avoid damp, sticky foods like melons, kiwis, rhubarb, artichokes, winter squashes, cucumbers, zucchini, sweet potatoes, nuts, cheeses, sour cream, yogurt, oatmeal, tofu and soy products, and cream pies. Follow a kapha reducing food plan.

Externally, you can apply a chest salve of eucalyptus and menthol or camphor. These salves usually come in a beeswax. Rub them on the chest region. You can even inhale vapors from an oil diffuser such as mints, eucalyptus, camphor, or calamus. A dry warm climate such as Arizona is ideal. If you live in a cold damp climate, then use dehumidifiers in your home year round, especially during the humid seasons. Try to sauna every now and then to help dry out the respiratory passages. Some medicated herbal oils (nasaya) dropped with a dropper and inhaled up the nasal passages are good to keep the passages clear such as vegetable oil with ginger powder. Even a salt nasal wash done daily, is helpful. Smoking dry type herbs are helpful. Try sage, mints, cornsilk, coltsfoot, mullein, or horehound.

7) Back Pain

Cause: There are many different types of back pain and causes. Assuming you have no misalignment in the spine, or have not been in an accident or fall recently, in which case chiropractic care might be the better option, the cause is probably metabolic or due to stress. Anything internal can cause back pain, such as: a weak kidney condition, stress/muscle tension, osteoporosis, osteoarthritis, cancer, disintegrating discs, bulging swollen discs pressing on the nerves, or simply inflammation.

General kapha type back pain usually feels like a low grade but constant dull achy pain that worsens with lack of movement, or is worse first thing in the morning. The person will also feel lethargic in the morning and may be overweight. Pain will diminish with increased movement, circulation, dryness, and cooling substances. In this case, the pain is most likely to be due to excess heat, congestion, water retention or stagnation in that region.

Pitta type back pain usually feels like a strong, burning type pain. Sometimes the pain can feel like throbbing pain, but not necessarily burning pain. Other symptoms of heat in the body will usually be present, such as a red tongue, strong thirst and hunger, feeling hot often, a red facial complexion, etc. Acidic, heating, and spicy foods will make it flare up or become worse.

Vata type pain can feel like dull achy pain, or sharp pain, depending on the severity of the inflammation present. The pain will improve with moisture and coolness in the diet. The pain may travel around from place to place.

Back pain caused from muscle spasms, will be relieved by hot compresses or warm baths. A stress reduction program is mandatory for preventing this type of problem. Under stress, some people subconsciously tense their back muscles causing the muscles to cramp up.

Treatment: For vata back pain: Follow a vata reducing diet, but emphasize the cooling foods: cucumbers, avocado, zucchini, green beans, okra, asparagus, sweet potatoes, winter squashes, purple grapes, watermelon, honeydew, vanilla ice cream, milk, cottage cheese, white rice, and even soda. Avoid hot spices! Try either bala, Solomon's seal, or licorice root (2-3) capsules three times a day in combination with anti-inflammatory herbs: golden seal, gentian, or neem. Use the latter herbs in smaller doses. 1-2 tablespoons of castor oil will also help lubricate the system, keep the muscles flexible and reverse constipation and dryness in the tissues. Vitamin C and the herb amalaki are also good. For pain try the Indian herb jatamansi. If you have access to a hot tub, use it! If not, take hot baths frequently, since the heat helps muscles relax. You can even apply a ginger compress to the area of pain. To do this grate a small grapefruit size ball of ginger root and tie it up in a cheesecloth. Squeeze the juice out into a large soup pan filled 2/3 full of water on the stove, then drop the ball into the pot. Heat the pot up until very hot but not burning to the skin. Dip a small towel into the ginger bath, wring it out and apply directly to the site of pain. Place another towel over it to hold the heat in. Repeat these steps when the towel becomes cool. Try this for 15 minutes. Follow up with tiger balm rubbed and left on the area of pain. Get more rest but do plenty of yoga or stretching type exercises.

For pitta inflammatory type pain: Follow a pitta reducing diet, avoiding hot spices, vinegar, lemons, grapefruit, too many tomatoes or anything acidic. Try 1-2 capsules of jatamansi or white willow bark for pain. (Avoid willow bark if allergic to aspirin.) A tea made from skullcap, catnip, hops and peppermint will help both pain and inflammation at the same time. Bala, shatavari, licorice, and marshmallow root will mildly help sooth inflammation, cool, and moisten. Bhumy amalaki, dandelion, aloe vera, golden seal, and neem will more strongly put out fire/inflammation, along with Chinese herbal formulas for clearing heat. Avoid using any of these herbs while taking prescription or over the counter pain relievers that are blood thinning. Emphasize cool showers and baths, and apply coconut oil to the area of pain along with ice packs.

For kapha back pain: Follow a kapha-pitta reducing diet and lifestyle, especially avoiding yogurt, sour cream, cheese, citrus, tomatoes, spicy foods, and heavy foods like oatmeal which promote water retention, mucus, congestion, and heat. Exercise frequently!
Try bitter herbs, and mild diuretics to break up congestion, decrease fats, decrease heat, decrease water, and stiffness. Bitters are: aloe, dandelion, neem, gentian root, golden seal, and bhumy amalaki. Some diuretics include: dandelion, uva ursi, cornsilk, and cleavers. Chicory grain coffee is not bad as a beverage, along with peppermint or chamomile tea. Even soda can help. For actual pain relieving herbs, use skullcap, hops, catnip, white willow bark, or jatamansi. Avoid willow bark if allergic to aspirin.

8) Bone Spurs/Bunions on the Feet

Cause: Bone spurs or bunions are really bone protrusions and result from a lack of calcium in the diet and/or an overall acid condition. Pitta people are most susceptible to these, but all types can develop them. When the human body becomes too acidic, it makes balance by releasing alkaline minerals from the bones such as calcium to neutralize the acid. During this process of transportation, the minerals can become lodged in places they do not belong such as on the feet or in the breast tissue. Human pH must be slightly alkaline to survive (7.4). The body re-alkalizes itself through the buffer system. This condition usually means that your diet is too acidic, and/or your body type is naturally more acidic than most people's. Unfortunately, only surgery can remove them from the body. All one can do is prevent them from reoccurring.

Treatment: Reduce or eliminate acidic foods such as tomatoes, coffee, vinegar, lemons, limes, grapefruit, papaya, kiwis, rhubarb, berries/strawberries, yogurt, sour cream, buttermilk, pickles, alcohol, cranberries, green apples, and consume these fruits only if sweet, ripe, or swimming in sugar syrup: apples, pears, oranges, pineapple, mangoes, grapes, plums, cherries, apricots, prunes, blueberries, cantaloupe, coconut, dates, figs, bananas, peaches. Basically, eat more pitta reducing foods that decrease acid production in the body. Try 1200 mg cal/mag a day to prevent this problem from worsening. Make sure the calcium and magnesium is in a 2:1 ratio. The calcium should be about

1200 mg. Also include 400 IU of vitamin D. The magnesium and vitamin D helps the body absorb the calcium. Boron is not a bad mineral to look for in your calcium formula, because it also helps increase calcium's absorption in the body. Foods that are either high in calcium or that buffer acidity are: kale, collards, broccoli, bok choy, okra, carrots and juice, beans/legumes especially soy products, tahini/sesame seeds, almonds, milk, ice cream, cottage cheese, ricotta cheese, figs, prunes, blackstrap molasses, sardines, scallops, lobster, red sweet apples, pears, sweet purple grapes, melons, cauliflower, dates, white potatoes. Herbs that are either high in calcium or buffer acidity are shatavari, Solomon's seal, comfrey root, licorice root, fo-ti, slippery elm, dandelion, neem, gentian root, golden seal, red clover. Seek professional advice when considering comfrey, because this herb can be toxic in large or too frequent doses and can cause liver failure. Kaphas can try the lighter anti-acid herbs such as: turmeric, aloe vera, neem, dandelion, golden seal, or red clover. A tea made from peppermint, mullein, dandelion, lemongrass, and lemon balm is also helpful.

9) Bronchitis

Cause: This is often a pitta-related illness and kapha, kapha-pittas, pittas, and pitta-vatas are most susceptible to it, although anyone can develop it. It is basically an inflammation/infection of the bronchi. In any case, spicy foods, alcohol, coffee, yogurt, cheese, sour cream, and other heating substances, should be strictly avoided. Cooling foods should be emphasized, depending on the body type, such as: kale, collards, peas, green beans, okra, lettuce, spinach, cucumbers, avocado, asparagus, red apples, pears, purple grapes, dates, watermelon, honeydew, coconut, figs, milk, vanilla ice cream, and even soda.

Treatment: For the kapha, kapha-pitta type person, bitters such as turmeric, dandelion, bhumy amalaki, neem, echinacea, gentian, golden seal, aloe vera will help fight infection and inflammation as they are antibiotic. Try 1 capsule 3 –4 times a day, depending on your weight and the severity of your condition. Never stay on these herbs indefinitely. If you have much damp mucus associated with this, then use drying and expectorant herbs such as vasaka, mullein, red raspberry leaf, cornsilk, agrimony, and peppermint. Cooling diuretics will also help decrease any water in the lungs such as dandelion, cleavers, or uva ursi.

A pitta, pitta-vata predominate person with this medical condition and dryness in the lungs, can use cooling moistening herbs with the bitters, such as marshmallow, licorice, shatavari or Solomon's seal combined with golden seal or neem. If the pitta person has heavy, abundant, thick mucus with yellow or green color, mullein, red raspberry leaf or peppermint tea will help cool and dry the respiratory system. One to two 1/2 teaspoons of vasaka a day will help breathing also.

10) Candida (yeast infections)

Cause: In my opinion, most yeast infections are caused from excess pitta in the system, or too much acidity and heat. Kapha and kapha-pitta type people tend towards excessive dampness, heat, and acidity internally (a perfect medium for yeast to grow in, like mold growing in a damp basement). Pitta people are naturally sensitive to sour and fermented foods and develop candida because these foods in their diets tend to stagnate and ferment in the gut. Vaginal yeast infections often come with a burning sensation. Vatas often experience dryness, along with infection, hence complain of vaginal itching during a yeast infection. Finally, anyone who uses large amounts of antibiotics and birth control pills is at some risk for developing candida, because these prescription drugs destroy the good bacteria in the gut, allowing for the overgrowth of yeast. However, the key to permanently eliminating yeast overgrowth is not rotation diets, yeast-free, or sugar free diets, but decreasing pitta/acid/heat! And sugar is both cooling and a natural anti-acid!

Treatment: For the kapha damp type: Avoid/cut back spicy food, acidic foods, and damp foods such as winter squashes, bananas, kiwis, lemons, limes, grapefruit, yogurt, sour cream, cheese, nuts, tomatoes, zucchini, parsnips, artichokes, milk, ice cream, cucumbers, olives, pickles, too much wheat and rice products, oatmeal, yams, pumpkin, tofu, oranges, and pineapple. Keep your food dry. Herbs for yeast infections and water retention include: uva ursi, golden seal, dandelion, gentian root, neem, and echinacea. Occasional salt baths, and dry saunas will help pull excess water out of your system. Fill a bathtub with warm water up to your hip level while dumping in 5 beer mugs full of water softener salt. The salt in the tub will be greater in concentration than that in your body creating an osmosis effect and pull the water out. You need to sit in a tub for 30 minutes for this to occur.

For the sour sensitive pitta person: avoid fermented foods, sour foods, sour beverages and spices such as garlic, grapefruit, tomatoes, kiwis, cranberry juice, pickles, coffee, black tea, soy sauce, miso, tempeh, wine, beer, papaya, rhubarb, strawberries, buttermilk, sour cream, hard cheeses, sour fruits and juices, lemonade, veggie and soy burgers, yogurt, and acidophilus. Follow a naturally sweet pitta tasting diet. Bitter herbs will regulate your digestive tract, and kill off yeast such as aloe vera gel, neem, turmeric, dandelion, red chicory, golden seal, echinacea, or bhumy amalaki. These can be taken as is, or with heavier more moistening herbs like shatavari, marshmallow, or licorice root. I have found that in pitta predominant type people, acidophilus and yogurt makes their condition worse so I recommend strictly avoiding them!

For the vata type: Emphasize in your diet milk, ice cream, cottage cheese, red grapes, pears, coconut, dates, figs, melons, zucchini, cucumbers, zucchini, green beans, okra, avocado, winter squashes, and asparagus. Acidophilus capsules or in liquid form are okay for a vata. Herbal formulas should contain: marshmallow, licorice or shatavari with golden seal or neem.

11) Canker Sores

Cause: Canker sores are little mouth ulcers. They simply mean that your system is currently too acidic and aggravated by too many sour foods or spices. Again, this is a common complaint in pitta predominant people. I strongly suggest avoiding vitamin C as it is very acidic.

Treatment: Avoid sour, fermented and spicy foods such as grapefruit, lemons, limes, rhubarb, strawberries, sour fruits and sour juices, yogurt, sour cream, too many tomatoes, pickles, alcohol, coffee, green apples, cranberry juice, and vinegar. Neutralize the acid in your system by consuming more pitta reducing foods, as these buffer acidity. Ice cream and milk, along with purple grapes, red sweet apples, dates, broccoli, and kale do this nicely. For two weeks try one of the following depending on your body type:

For vata, vata-pitta, and pitta-vata types try one of the following: 1/4 tsp. or 1 capsule of a combination of shatavari, bala, or Solomon's seal with guduchi or neem three times a day. You could also try pouring 1 cup of hot water over 1/2 teaspoon of fennel powder, and 1/4 teaspoon turmeric powder. Sweeten with sugar and drink twice a day. All these combinations are anti-acid. A calcium/magnesium tablet will also help stop acid production in your gut by buffering it.

For pittas try a combination of Solomon's seal, shatavari, bala, or licorice root with turmeric, dandelion, bhumy amalaki, or neem.

For kapha or kapha-pitta types try one of the following: gentian root, dandelion, golden seal, neem, or turmeric.

12) The Common Cold

Cause: There are many viruses in the atmosphere that cause a person to develop a cold. Some people always seem to "catch" one because their immune system is weaker than that of the others. Therefore, strengthening immune function by strengthening your constitution will help, as well as taking immune stimulating herbs for your particular body type and eating the right diet. In addition to that, people develop specific symptoms unique to their body's current state of imbalance. For example, excessive dryness in the system can cause a dry cough, excessive heat and or acidity can cause a sore throat, etc. When treating a cold, always look at the specific symptoms you have. Is the cough dry or is there a rattling sound, and is there much sputum, or is there a sore throat and how severe is the inflammation? Are the sinuses stuffed and if so, does any mucus run out, what color is the mucus, how thick or thin is it, and do your nasal passages burn or feel dry?

Generally speaking, the kapha cold will have heavy, abundant, thick, white mucus. Kapha-pitta will have green or yellow streaks in the sputum, indicating internal infection. The cough will sound strong and forceful, or a rattling sound might be heard. The vata cold/cough will usually come with a dry hacking cough, laryngitis, dry nostrils, very little mucus, maybe a thin clear runny type nasal drip, a dry itchy throat. The pitta cold will have symptoms of infection or inflammation such as blood or yellow streaked mucus and sputum, a sore inflamed throat, a fever, or burning nasal passages.

In my opinion, the other main reason for developing colds is not compensating for the changes in the climate by adjusting your diet to fit the seasons and climate influence. While the cold air is not a virus and does not cause a cold directly, it can weaken you as an external pathogen. This means you need to compensate by dressing more warmly, eating warming foods and beverages, and adding more spices to your diet in cold weather. Use common sense. For example, reduce your consumption of ice cream and salads in winter, and include more soups, stews, and hot chocolate. Read more about this under my section on seasonal cooking and eating.

Treatment: Vata immune tonics are: ashwagandha, licorice, shatavari, slippery elm, Solomon's seal, marshmallow, wild yam, codonopsis, ginseng, amalaki, hawthorn berries, rehmannia root, astragalus, vitamin C, zinc, oily vitamins like A, D, and E, garlic, fo-ti, kapikacchu, bala, and the Japanese kudzu root and umeboshi plums. These herbs and supplements strengthen qi (your vitality, life force, or immune system). Vata reducing foods will also help the immune system. For dryness and congestion in the nasal passages try several capsules a day of licorice root, Solomon's seal, or marshmallow root along with a ginger if you are cold. Ginger and licorice tea (4 times as much licorice than ginger) is good, or a tea made from: comfrey, licorice, fennel, eucalyptus and orange peel. Lemon and sugar is excellent for the vata cold as it is moistening. For a dry scratchy throat, try slippery elm dissolved in the mouth and moistening herbs like 2 capsules 2-3 times a day of licorice, Solomon's seal, or shatavari with cinnamon or cardamom. Look for warm moist formulas, unless there are heat signs present. In general, vatas tend to have the weakest immune systems, but anyone can have a strong constitution and wreck it.

Pitta immune tonics are marshmallow, shatavari, Solomon's seal, bala, kappicacchu, slippery elm, and licorice. These herbs are cooling and moistening and help lubricate dry, inflamed mucous membranes. Where there is infection/inflammation such as in a bad sore throat, bitter tonics help such as echinacea, bhumy amalaki, neem, aloe vera gel, gentian, and golden seal. Bitters should only be used during the duration of an infection, then withdrawn. Even a gargle can be made out of 1 teaspoon of turmeric and honey, equal parts, in a glass of warm water, used several times throughout the day for a sore throat. Salads, vanilla ice cream, milk, red or purple grapes are excellent food/beverage choices. Follow a pitta reducing diet to maintain and strengthen your health. A tea can be brewed from: licorice, comfrey, and peppermint. Just plain mullein and mint tea is good if there is also a lot of heavy damp type mucus and inflammation, as these herbs are drying. Vasaka powder can also be taken, such as 1/4 teaspoon two to three times a day or in capsule form, for damp type mucus.

Kapha immune tonics are golden seal, aloe vera, neem, gentian, and echinacea, for inflammation or infection. If no inflammation or infection exists, but there is much mucus as in a heavy cough, try garlic, ginger, mullein, red raspberry leaf, dandelion leaf, pipplai, trikatu, cinnamon, clove to break it up. Try several of these combined in their powdered form with honey as a paste, in capsule form or as a tea formula. A good tea combination is: mullein, elecampane, thyme, bayberry bark, sage, eucalyptus, and ephedra. Use 1 teaspoon of herbs per cup of water. Use ephedra in tiny doses, since it is a very strong stimulant. Do not take it if you have heart trouble, high blood pressure, anxiety or other nervous system disorders such as insomnia. Discontinue its use if you experience hyperactivity, rapid pulse, insomnia, nervousness, or heart palpitations. Strain and drink, sweeten with honey. Vasaka can also be taken in equal amounts with pipplai or trikatu and honey such as 1/4 to 1/2 teaspoon twice a day. The macrobiotic lotus root tea is good for drying up mucus. A chest salve of eucalyptus and menthol, or a ginger or mustard and flour paste can be applied to the chest. Be careful to mix the mustard with some flour since the mustard can burn the skin. Spicy teas are great for the kapha cold.

13) Cold Hands and Feet/Feeling Cold All the Time

Cause: Another sign of coldness in the body is frequent "clear" urination. Also, your tongue may be pale in color (a normal tongue is pink), you may sleep curled up in a ball at night in bed, and desire extra clothing such as sweaters and socks. You may have no thirst and a pale complexion, cold hands and feet, little or no perspiration, which are all signs of coldness in the body according to Chinese medicine. Pure vata and pure kapha types develop this condition more easily, along with dual doshic (mixed) types such as vata-pittas and kapha-pittas.

Treatment: Ingest more substances that have a warming effect on the body. Below is a list. Pick those that you prefer the taste of, or those that are more suited to your body type. Also, dress in layers and abundantly. Keep the temperature in your home higher. Avoid air conditioning and drafts. Wear hats, gloves or mittens in the winter, if you live in the northeast or northwest. Practice some color therapy to make you visually and psychologically feel warmer. Choose reds, yellows, gold, orange, black, brown. Avoid rooms that are blue and white. If you are a kapha type, sauna once in a while. Sunbathe with sunscreen. Do aerobic exercise like tennis or jogging or biking to heat up and make sweat. When you eat, emphasize cooked foods over raw. Emphasize more warming spices in your diet. Avoid too many salads, ice cream, tofu, soda and juices. Even watch the herbal teas you are drinking. Some have a cooling effect on the body such as chamomile, peppermint, and licorice. A cup of hot chocolate in the winter is more warming, or warmed cow's or soy milk with cinnamon. Coffee is very heating and excellent for kapha types or ginger and spicy based teas.

Warm foods/substances: bananas, bell peppers, green grapes, peaches, apricots, cantaloupe, cherries, cranberries, brown lentils, oats, brown rices, nuts, chocolate, eggs, oranges, pineapple, plums, mangoes, papaya, plantains, tomatoes, cheese, yogurt, molasses, carrots, beets, seafood, poultry, beef, globe artichokes, radishes, onions, garlic, Brussels sprouts, corn on cob, black olives, soy sauce, miso, ginger, cinnamon, cardamom, cloves, allspice, orange peel, basil, oregano, bay leaf, rosemary, thyme, sage, chili powder, chilies, horseradish, curry, black pepper, sea salt, sea vegetables, sesame seeds, burdock root, pumpkin, mushrooms, marjoram, paprika, turmeric. The bottom line is, cook with spices. Spices heat the body up as well as promote circulation. Pick either mild or the hotter spices depending on your tastes and body system. If chili powder puts your mouth on fire, gives you some loose stools, or diarrhea, then choose the milder warm spices like basil, cinnamon, etc. Hotter is not always necessary. Listen to your body.

14) Colitis and/or Chronic Diarrhea

Cause: Sour, fermented, damp, juicy, sweet, and very strong spicy foods and beverages cause this condition. Excess spicy foods and strong spices increase the peristaltic motion of the intestinal tract, pushing foods through too fast. Moistening foods, including sweet as well as sour foods, soften and loosen stools as these foods are damp. Pitta types and pitta/kaphas have the greatest tendency towards diarrhea or loose stools due to their damp nature.

In Chinese medicine, diarrhea it is seen as a damp condition of the spleen. Other dampness symptoms that may be present are: a sticky or greasy coated tongue, excessive saliva, nausea, lack of hunger, lack of thirst, thick white vaginal discharge (if you are female), and possibly a heavy feeling in the legs and arms or edema.

Treatment: Avoid taking digestive enzyme supplements or acidophilus as they worsen this problem. Avoid sour, heavy, spicy, and fermented foods: grapefruit, papaya, grapes, bananas, lemons, limes, kiwis, pineapple, orange juice, melons, tomatoes, winter squashes, zucchini, yogurt, sour cream, buttermilk, cottage cheese, oatmeal, coffee, alcohol, tempeh, miso, soy sauce, sourdough bread, mustard, garlic, chilies, horseradish, ginger, curry, salsa, ketchup, pickles, and too much black pepper. Try 1/4 tsp. 3 times a day of equal parts of cumin, punarnava, and coriander with meals. Also try: red raspberry leaf, peppermint, mullein, dandelion, and agrimony tea (two cups a day in place of your usual beverages), or a combination of chamomile, thyme, mint, lemongrass, cleavers, and dandelion tea. The Ayurvedic herbs arjuna, musta, and ashoka in capsule form, also bind stools. Natural chicory grain coffees such as kaffree roma, pero or caffix are excellent. Black tea is an astringent, and will help stop diarrhea by also binding the stools. Gentian root extract is an excellent herb for this condition too. You can take around 1/2 teaspoon twice a day with meals for a few weeks. There are many excellent Chinese formulas and herbs to stop this condition such as those containing magnolia bark, alisma, atractylodes, bupleurum, poria, ammomum, saussurea, ailanthes. Basically any formula that is overall drying will stop diarrhea, including diuretic herbs like uva ursi, dandelion, or cornsilk. If you have a tendency towards dryness in your system, but temporarily have loose stools, pick an herb formula that is not totally drying. Look for one that contains a mixture of drying and moistening herbs such as the Chinese traditional formula six gentleman.

15) Conjunctivitis

Cause: This is due to high pitta in the system. Conjunctivitis is an infection or inflammation of the mucous membranes of the eyelids and eye. Characteristically, the eyes become pink and hence the nickname pink eye.

Treatment: You can try aloe vera gel dropped gently into the eyes, or brew a tea of chrysanthemum or chamomile flowers (1 teaspoon herbs per cup hot water). Make sure the tea is cool before applying the drops to the eyes. Internally, chrysanthemum can be taken or you can try dandelion, neem, bhumy amalaki, or use an echinacea and golden seal extract. They are natural antibiotics. Be cautious because they are bitter herbs. If you are a vata person, consider taking them in a formula with heavier, anti-inflammatory herbs such as shatavari, marshmallow or licorice root to prevent vata health problems from developing.

16) Constipation (chronic)

Cause: Chronic constipation has to due with either a lack of moisture in the body, too many hard and astringent substances in the diet binding the stool, lack of whole grains/dietary fiber, or not enough spice in your cooking to increase the peristaltic motion of the digestive tract. In short, you may be too internally dried up. Just drinking more water doesn't always reverse this. Your diet needs to include more moisture increasing foods, as well as softer, slightly oily, and spicy foods. Obviously, this is the opposite condition of diarrhea or colitis. Look under that section to get a better understanding of this cause. Chronic constipation occurs more often in vata type people who tend towards dryness. Kapha people or mixed types can also experience this to a lesser extent.

Treatment for the vata type: Sour, sweet, juicy, and spicy foods and beverages relieve this condition. Triphala is a good Indian herb consisting of three tropical fruits. One can try 2 capsules at bedtime with a glass of orange or pineapple juice. In addition to this he/she can add 1-2 tablespoons of castor oil, or simply add castor oil to a glass of warm milk with ginger and sugar. In extreme cases, use buttermilk. Also try 2-3 capsules 2-3 times a day of licorice root, rehmannia root, fo-ti, or Solomon's seal. You may also want to follow a vata reducing diet, as well as eating plenty of whole grains such as brown rice, oatmeal and whole wheat bread. Yogurt with ginger powder, lemon juice, or just fruit and sugar added is good too. Tomato sauce is excellent for relieving chronic constipation as well as red grape juice. Hingwastak, asafoetida, garlic, and ajwain seeds are good strong vata spices for helping constipation.

For the vata –pitta or pitta-vata person, simply taking yin tonic herbs such as licorice root, marshmallow or Solomon's seal and drinking more fruit juices like orange juice, pineapple, grape, and coconut are helpful. Cooked garlic, extra salt, black pepper, chili powder, and cinnamon in cooking, may be stimulating enough.

For the kapha type - include hot spices in your diet. Try pungent spicy herbs such as ginger, trikatu, garlic, pipplai, cinnamon, black pepper. Aloe vera and senna are laxatives that can be taken temporarily (but do not take both at the same time). Do not take senna for extended periods of time and research its cautions before using. Include plenty of high fiber foods such as peaches and high fiber cereals.

17) Cracking in the Joints/Spine

Cause: Your synovial fluid has dried up some, or you have a deterioration of cartilage in the knees. The knees or spine may crack like popcorn when you bend them. Usually this is more common in vata people or vata-pitta people, although anyone can develop this. Pitta types can develop cracking and dryness in the joints also.

Treatment: You need to moisten your body internally by ingesting more foods that do just that (such as vata reducing foods or plasma increasing foods). If the cause is a loss of cartilage, supply your body with more vata decreasing, heavier foods and herbs. Foods which tend to be more moistening, and help build plasma are: lemons, limes, grapefruit, coconut, red grapes, bananas, melons, plums, oranges, pineapple, mangoes, peaches, zucchini, cucumbers, summer squashes, winter squashes, pumpkin, tomatoes/ketchup, globe artichokes, sweet juices, yogurt, sour cream, ice cream, wheat, oatmeal, brown and white rices, tofu, seafood, and dark meat poultry. Moistening herbs include: fo-ti, kapikacchu, Solomon's seal, fennel, licorice root, shatavari, or marshmallow. Vitamin C, triphala, amalaki, and hawthorn berries help the body build moisture and prevent cartilage deterioration in vata types as well. Oily foods such as vegetable oil in the diet or nuts are good. You can also use oil externally by massaging the entire body with it. Good heavy vata reducing oils for this condition are sesame, almond, castor, and coconut oil. Regular baths, oatmeal baths, and swimming in fresh water are suggested.

18) Dandruff

Cause: This is simply caused from too much internal dryness, or too much heat in the body burning up your fluids which causes the skin on the scalp to dry out. Many companies try to sell you specialty shampoos to alleviate dandruff, but in reality they aren't that effective because dryness, flaking, and itching of the scalp is an internal problem! If you purchase a shampoo, look for one with fatty substances such as coconut or wheat germ oil in it, or one that contains fruity substances.

Treatment: Moisten up your diet and drink plenty of sweet or sweet-sour juices. Eat more vata reducing foods. Avoid dry beans, herbal teas, popcorn, corn chips, pretzels, too much cabbage, cauliflower, dry fruits, and salads. Externally you can rub almond, coconut, olive, or sesame oil into the scalp. Internally try 2 capsules 2-3 times a day of shatavari, licorice, marshmallow, Solomon's seal, kapikacchu, or fo-ti.

If there is too much heat in your body (red tongue, hot flashes, night sweats, feeling too warm during the day or night, flushed face), your diet should temporarily contain plenty of cooling foods and beverages to reverse this. Emphasize plenty of salads, zucchini, broccoli, cauliflower, cabbage, asparagus, green beans, peas, white rice, wheat products, milk, ice cream, okra, kale, collards, yellow summer squash, cucumbers, apples, pears, purple grapes, berries, melons, dates, figs, and/or coconut. Many pitta reducing herbs are cooling. Research them first. Coconut oil externally on the scalp is good.

19) Depression

Cause: There are two main causes for depression: physical and environmental. Environmental or relationship circumstances can contribute to depression, along with past circumstances/issues. Professional counseling will help in these cases. However, see section 8 of this book for more ideas. In my opinion, there is only one true physical cause for depression: excess qi or being way too grounded. Lethargy, afternoon napping, excess weight gain, edema, and trouble waking up in the morning are associated with this pattern. Generally, kapha types or the obese will have depression due to excess, and vatas and vata-pittas will have depression purely for psychological reasons. kapha types can also have depression for external reasons.

Treatment: For the physical kapha type: literally lift your emotional state over a period of months by lightening up your diet and lifestyle. Follow a kapha or kapha-pitta reducing diet like the ones listed at the beginning of this book. Get regular aerobic exercise to add more air and ether back into your system, stimulate metabolism, and lift the emotional state. Weight loss will help reverse physical depression. Herbally try 1/4 teaspoon three times a day of brahmi and shankpushpi, or 1 capsule of brahmi and ginko 3 times a day. Also try 2 cups a day of tea made from sage, basil, sassafras, and peppermint. Coffee is a great beverage in this case. You might also want to take 1/4 cup of aloe vera gel internally in the morning for a few weeks and 1 capsule (1/4th tsp.) of a combination of ginger, punarnava, dandelion, coriander, and trikatu three times a day, or a formula made from equal parts ginger, cinnamon, dandelion, cleavers, and peppermint, provided you have no heartburn or ulcers. If water retention exists, try uva ursi as a diuretic. All of these herbs will lift “kapha” type depression because they help break down tissue, dry out the body, and stimulate the body and nervous system. Excess kapha causes depression because extra dampness in the tissues and excess fat, pull the body "down," making the individual too grounded, lethargic, and tired. The nerves become dulled making the kapha individual not able to think clearly. For aromatherapy, use stimulating scents such as cinnamon, mint, camphor, juniper, musk, amber, or cedar. Use stimulating, fast rhythm, but also happy music, in your home, work, or car environment.

20) Dizziness

Cause and Treatment: This can indicate a serious medical problem. Please have your physician check it out. Low and high blood pressure, and epilepsy can cause this. (For blood pressure problems, look under those sections of this book in part 6.) Even water trapped in the ear canals from chronic sinus trouble, can cause dizziness. If all of the above are ruled out, sometimes a blood deficiency/anemic condition can cause it. (Look under anemia in section 6 of this book to treat it.) The other main cause of unexplained dizziness, according to Ayurveda, is high vata in the system (too much air-wind and ether trapped in the body). Follow my suggestions for a vata reducing diet in the beginning of this book. You can also take herbs that dispel wind and build vitality or "qi." They are: ginseng, ashwagandha, shatavari, licorice, Solomon's seal, fo-ti, kapikacchu, bala, the Indian tonic chywan prash, hawthorn berries, codonopsis root, rehmannia root, wild yam, and amalaki. Another action one can take, to reverse this condition, is to fill the ear canals completely with warm sesame oil. Let the oil sit for at least 5 minutes before expelling it from the ears. You may want to do this every day for a while.

21) Dry Skin and Hair

Cause: Basically, there are two causes for this: internal dryness or too much internal heat drying up the body's fluids including the moisture content of the hair and skin. Other symptoms of internal dryness are: a dry mouth, dry nostrils, dry lips, cracked hands, peeling of the skin on your body, no perspiration or very little of it.

Treatment: Consume more plasma increasing foods and beverages in your diet (rice, wheat, oatmeal, lemons, limes, grapefruit, kiwis, oranges, pineapple, mangoes, cantaloupe/melons, bananas, grapes, fresh figs, coconut, yams, winter squash, zucchini, cucumbers, tomatoes, artichokes, yogurt, milk, cottage cheese, sugar, maple syrup, sweet juicy juices, and sea salt. Follow more of a vata diet or emphasize more vata reducing foods. Vitamin C is excellent since it helps build collagen and draws in moisture. Try a 500 mg tablet once a day. Hawthorn berries and amalaki are other good sour herbs that help build plasma and collagen. Other moisture restoring herbs include: fo-ti, bala, licorice, Solomon's seal, shatavari, kapikacchu, marshmallow, and slippery elm. Lemonade, grape juice, orange juice, pineapple, and coconut milk are excellent ways to help replenish moisture quickly.

Externally, massage oils into the skin to seal the moisture in and further lubricate the skin (use heavy oils like coconut, olive, almond or sesame). Rub some of the oil into your scalp and let it soak in. To prevent premature wrinkling, wear sunscreen daily when outside for more than 10-15 minutes. Once or twice a day, apply skin creams that help rebuild collagen and moisturize. Make sure the cream contains Vitamin C, E, and retinyl A, as well as natural moisturizers like papaya, coca butter, coconut, cucumber, almond oil, or pineapple. A natural facial moisturizer can be made from mixing pineapple, avocado and banana in a blender. Leave on for 15-20 minutes before taking off. Regular baths in plain bathtub water, fresh lake or pond water are excellent for rehydrating the skin. The body will absorb a small amount of water through the skin. Try an oatmeal-oil bath. Place 1 cup of instant oats in a cheesecloth and tie shut with a rubber band. Drop this ball in the bathtub as it is filling with warm water. Rub sesame or almond oil all over your body and then sit in the tub for 20 minutes. Avoid using soap, as most kinds strip natural body oils. If you must, look for ones containing fatty oils and fruity substances such as oatmeal, coconut oil, goat's milk, and olive oil. Look for shampoos that contain also contain these substances. Shirodhara, an Ayurvedic warm oil treatment to the head and scalp, is very beneficial for this condition. This is done by pouring a continuous warm stream of oil over the forehead and scalp, hitting pressure points. The oil soaks into the scalp and forehead.

22) Edema

Cause: Edema is a serious medical condition that deserves the attention of a natural holistic practitioner and physician. Kapha predominant people are the most susceptible to developing this medical disorder because of their system's natural tendency to retain water. If too many watery/damp foods are eaten over a lifetime, they are at risk for developing edema. Sweet, salty, and sour type foods will cause this, or drinking too many fluids. One of the classic signs of a person who is consuming too many fluids, is puffiness under the lower eyelids. Edema can also be caused from: weak kidneys, a weakness of the spleen/digestive system or a problem with the lungs or heart. Sometimes, but not always, the area of the edema will be a clue as to the cause of the edema. Generally, edema below the waist in the legs and ankles is due to weak kidney function. When the swelling is in the fingers and hands, most often the spleen/digestive system is involved and the digestive system must be balanced. The spleen/digestive system also is partially responsible for regulating the circulation of fluids throughout the body, especially in the hands. In all cases, the root cause must be treated. If extreme internal coldness over a long period of time has caused a weakening of the kidneys' ability to remove water, then the focus of treatment must be to restore internal heat to the body, particularly the kidney region. In Chinese medicine, that condition is called kidney yang deficiency, and anybody can develop it. In kidney yang deficiency, the following symptoms are usually present: cold hands and feet, lack of thirst, frequent profuse, clear urination, nighttime urination, lower back pain, edema in the legs or ankles, and possible fatigue.

Treatment: For kapha edema, emphasize kapha reducing foods that are naturally drier. Avoid heavy, damp food as much as possible such as winter squashes, melons, cucumbers, coconut, grapefruit, lemons, limes, oatmeal, tomatoes, bananas, sugary drinks, tofu, oranges, pineapple, artichokes, and nuts. Uva ursi, shilajit, parsley, cleavers, juniper berries, cornsilk, chickweed, dandelion, gokshura, and punarnava are all natural diuretics. A Chinese formula for temporarily draining dampness in the body can contain: alisma, cinnamon bark, atractylodes, and poria. If your mouth starts becoming dry, you are taking too much. To strengthen the kidneys in cases of kidney yang deficiency, use warming, light, and drying kidney tonic herbs beneficial to the kapha person. Some of them are: teasel root, shilajit, morinda root, eucommia bark, cinnamon, ginger, psoralea fruit, garlic, ajwain seeds, acrythranthes root, and angelica. Both acrythranthes and angelica have aspirin like/pain relieving properties, and are good especially for lower back pain associated with this condition. The majority of these herbs can be used in conduction with smaller amounts of the diuretic herbs: punarnava, gokshura, uva ursi, or parsley. For kidney yang deficiency, the formula, overall, should slant towards the warming side, keeping in mind that the underlying cause is coldness. A salt bath in your bathtub or ocean swim will help draw out water and strengthen the kidneys. Never take plain water baths for this condition. They will make it much worse. To do a salt bath, fill a tub with very warm water up to your hip level. Add 5 beer mugs of water softener salt crystals to the bath to dissolve. The salty water pulls the water out of your body by an osmosis process, provided your bath lasts 30 minutes. A sauna once a week is good also for pulling out moisture from the body. Saunas also strengthen the kidneys by drawing out heavy metals and acids from the body, thereby giving the kidneys a rest. Sauna until you sweat for a 2-3 minutes. One sauna a week is sufficient for kaphas. Avoid a sauna if you have dry deficiency type health problems, hypertension or any heart problems. Also read the recommendations in this book under cold hands and feet, but continue to avoid the damp foods as well.

For kidney yang deficiency in vata and vata-pitta types - use warming herbs, spices, and foods to dispel deep internal coldness in the kidney region and body. Some are: cotton root, ashwagandha, saw palmetto, garlic, cinnamon, astragalus root and seed, cornus fruit, Chinese ginseng, schisandra, cordyceps fungus, cynomorium stem, and cistanche stem. The Chinese classic formula rehmannia 8 is a great formula for kidney yang deficiency in a vata, vata-pitta, or pitta-vata type person, as vata body types tend to be internally dry and cold, but can nevertheless have edema due to weak kidney function. The kidney formula should be moistening as well as warming. Rehmannia 8 often contains cornus fruit, cooked rehmannia root, fuling, wild yam, poria, alisma and aconite or cinnamon bark to warm it. Pitta predominant people could benefit from a simple formula of cooked rehmannia root, or baked licorice with cinnamon or cardamom added to it.

23) Epstein-Barr Virus/Chronic Fatigue Syndrome

Cause: Epstein-Barr is a chronic immune disorder that also is often referred to as chronic fatigue syndrome. While the complications that can arise from this disorder are numerous, I strongly believe that the key to reversing this disorder is to strengthen the person's body constitution. When the constitution is weakened, the body is more susceptible to developing full blown Epstein-Barr symptoms. However, the symptoms will be slightly different in everyone depending on the nature of their body type and imbalance. The type of symptoms one develops is also related to which doshas are out of balance. For example, in pitta related Epstein-Barr, chronic sore throats and fevers are common symptoms, along with fatigue. With a vata imbalance, severe debilitating fatigue will be the most prevalent symptom along with deficiency type insomnia. The kapha type is more likely to experience muscle heaviness and stiffness, water retention, lethargy, fatigue due to excess, and a mind that just cannot remember thoughts very easily, or chronic “brain fog." Kapha-pitta predominant people can also develop the inflammatory symptoms that pitta predominant people do, if pitta dosha is out of balance.

Treatment: Follow the appropriate diet and lifestyle for your unique body type, take immune boosting herbs and supplements that match your body type, and try herbs that also reduce the imbalanced dosha or specific symptoms. (Look under the other diseases in this section of the book as to which herbs and treatments to follow for your symptoms.) For example, if you are a pitta predominate person with mostly pitta related symptoms, emphasize a pitta diet and lifestyle, take pitta immune boosting herb formulas such as those containing shatavari, licorice rehmannia, bala, ho-shou-wu, Solomon's seal or wild yam. Blood, liver, and/or lymph cleansers for toxic heat/infectious conditions are: red clover, guduchi, punarnava, milk thistle, neem, bhumy amalaki, echinacea, golden seal, and aloe vera. If you have chronic fevers and sore throats associated with this illness, take herbs that reduce inflammation, such as some of the ones just listed. Look up sore throats and use the appropriate foods until it disappears. If you have insomnia, look under insomnia for which herbs and foods to take, while simultaneously following the appropriate diet for you body type. If you have candida associated with your chronic fatigue syndrome, look under candida/yeast in this book.

Treatment for the vata predominant person with chronic fatigue should include tonic herb formulas that strengthen "qi," blood, the nerves, and so on. These formulas are heavy in their nature and build energy and stamina when there is much weakness and deficiency. The formulas should include: ho-shou-wu, codonopsis, ginseng, licorice root, rehmannia, ashwagandha, Solomon's seal, wild yam, bala, astragalus, longan fruit, red date, amalaki, Irish moss, or vamsha rochana. Since these are all quite heavy, make sure some lighter, slightly pungent herbs are added in small amounts to keep the formula from being too congesting. The combination of ashwagandha, bala, licorice, marshmallow, cinnamon, cardamom, and ginger is a good general formula, with the first four herbs in the greatest quantity. A good multi-vitamin and mineral formula wouldn't hurt either. If there is insomnia, follow the suggestions under insomnia in this book, and so on.

24) Fatigue

Cause: Fatigue can be due to many causes: low blood sugar(hypoglycemia), allergic reactions to particular foods, both short term acute and long term chronic sickness, anemic conditions, overwork, overexertion, excessive exercise, etc. However, pushing those factors aside, fatigue is usually rooted in one of two causes physiologically: excess or deficient "qi." In Ayurveda that would mean either high kapha or high vata. High kapha manifests itself as: weight gain, sluggishness, napping during the day, feeling lethargic in the morning where you need several cups of coffee to feel mentally alert, no motivation, depression. Fatigue, then, is due to excess: excess weight, excess dampness, excess congestion, a belief of Chinese medicine. The person is "too grounded." Grounded to the point where they have no energy.

Vata type deficiency fatigue, is the opposite condition. Hyperactivity may be present followed by extreme exhaustion, along with episodes of insomnia. Weight loss and anxiety tendencies may also accompany this. In this case, the individual does not have enough weight, muscle, lacks stamina, vitality, and may look a little frail. They lack abundance and hence need heavy nourishment. They may have other symptoms of deficiency in the body such as dizziness, a scanty menstrual period if they are female, and/or a soft or flabby tongue.

Pitta type individuals can have either types of fatigue. In this case, try the treatment under the deficiency type first, especially if you have no extra weight gain.

Treatment: For the excess kapha type reduce your consumption of heavy foods such as dairy products, melons, grapefruit, coconut, bananas, kiwis, lemons, limes, papaya, zucchini, winter squashes, oatmeal, tomatoes, yams, artichokes, parsnips, olives, sweet heavy pastries, nuts, soy products, tofu, and too many wheat products. Eat more corn tortillas/tacos, popcorn, rye breads, pretzels, crackers, corn chips, millet, dry cereals and granola. Emphasize lighter foods that literally "lift" the body and emotions. Select apples, pears, cranberries, peaches, apricots, prunes, raisins, berries, mangoes, plums, bell peppers, broccoli, cauliflower, cabbage, Brussels sprouts, leafy greens of all kinds, radishes, corn on cob, green and wax beans, mushrooms, onions, peas, potatoes, sprouts, legumes. Now and then, skipping a meal will make you feel lighter and more energized. Also, this type of person benefits the most from regular aerobic exercise that is a bit strenuous or of a fast tempo.

Stimulating herbs for this type are yang spices such as cooking with cinnamon, black pepper, chili powder, clove, ginger, garlic, cayenne, and bitter herbs such as aloe vera, dandelion, neem, bhumy amalaki, golden seal, burdock root, turmeric. Other Indian herbs to use are purified guggul, trikatu and pippali. If you are a person who gets headaches frequently or heartburn from the hot spices, try using milder ones like basil, mint, and sage. These three are stimulating to the nervous system. Brahmi and shank pushpi are two good Indian herbs for helping increase mental awareness. Coffee can be used as a temporary stimulant, because it reduces high kapha in the system. A chromium tablet as a supplement, is excellent for blood sugar problems. This supplement is also mildly stimulating.

In addition to this, wake up no later than 7:30 am. If you wake up later than this time, you feel more tired and lethargic. Try not to nap during the day and go to bed by 11pm. Include more mentally stimulating music as well as colors in your environment, and wear more reds, yellows, orange, and gold. Burn some stimulating incense such as cinnamon, cedar, or mental clearing aromas such as camphor, pine, eucalyptus, and sage.

For the deficient type of fatigue, the person needs nourishment! Take heavier vata reducing foods such as winter quashes, tomatoes, bananas, coconut, avocado, melons, mangoes, kiwi, papaya, oranges, pineapple, lemons, limes, dates, figs, cherries, red apples, apricots, grapes, plums, oat, wheat, and rice products, dairy foods, eggs, nuts, meats, more soy foods like tempeh, tofu, soy dogs and burgers, chocolate, summer squashes and sweet potatoes. For herbs try one or a combination of the following for four to twelve weeks: fo-ti, licorice, ginseng, shatavari, ashwagandha, cooked or raw rehmannia root, marshmallow, kapikacchu, Solomon's seal, codonopsis. Since these herbs are heavy, you might want to add a pinch of cinnamon, ginger, or cardamom to them or look for formulas that are mixed. Try 2 capsules of the formula 3 times a day or 1/2 tsp. 2 times a day. (Do not use ashwagandha, or ginseng if you have a history of menstrual irregularities, irritability, anger, migraine headaches, hot flashes, hypertension, or any pitta related problems.) Sea vegetables such as kelp, Irish moss, hijiki, and arame are excellent for a vata person suffering from chronic fatigue because they are very high in minerals. A good multi-vitamin and mineral formula may be a boost. Amino acids by tablet or protein shakes made from whey, egg whites, or soy protein are helpful here also, especially when there is muscle degeneration and emaciation. For an vata energizing shake, try 1 cup of milk blended with a banana, 1 egg, 1 teaspoon of vanilla, and a tablespoon of protein powder and spirulina. Aromatherapy for you may include scents of oranges, lemons, citrus as these are stimulating. Also reduce the amount of aerobic exercise and sexual activity you engage in, as these can drain the body. Try to get more rest and not over-exert yourself.

25) Fibromyalgia

Cause: Fibromyalgia is a pitta disorder. The number one chief complaint all fibromyalgia patients have is inflammatory type pain. Although other symptoms can accompany this disorder, inflammation is predominant. Inflammation is caused by excessive heat in the body. Think of your body as literally having too much "fire" in the muscle tissues and joints. People with a lot of pitta in their makeup, are at greatest risk for developing this painful disorder. Spicy foods, alcohol, coffee, garlic, and too many "heating" foods cause this in them.

Treatment: Emphasize cooling, anti-inflammatory, pitta-reducing foods and substances, these included: kale, collards, spinach, lettuce, cucumbers, peas, cabbage, green beans, asparagus, zucchini, okra, avocado, broccoli, cauliflower, white potatoes, white sugar, soda, vanilla ice cream, milk, tofu, red sweet apples, pears, red grapes, dates, coconut, figs, watermelon, honeydew, and white rice. Many good Chinese formulas to treat this are referred to as "purge fire" or "clear heat" formulas. Western and Indian herbs to try are: golden seal, neem, dandelion, mints, bhumy amalaki, gentian root, and aloe vera gel.

26) Frequent Urination (overactive bladder)

Cause: If no urinary tract infection is present, you are not taking prescription diuretics, and no tumor exists on or near the bladder, then the cause might simply be due to internal coldness in your bladder. When the body is internally cold, it tries to warm up by expelling more water in the form of urine since water cools the system down. Again, look for other symptoms of a cold condition such as a pale colored tongue, no thirst, little or no perspiration, cold hands and feet, sleeping in a curled position, desiring extra clothing, a pale face/complexion, frequent and clear colored urination, urine dribbling, and general intolerance to the cold weather. If this condition persists, it can turn into what is known as in Chinese medicine - kidney yang deficiency. Edema in the ankles and legs is also one of the telltale signs of kidney yang deficiency when the other above mentioned cold signs are also present. If this is the case, read the advice given under the section on the kidneys (treating kidney yang deficiency), found earlier in this book, and also read the section on how to treat edema.

Last, chronic anxiety can cause an overactive bladder. Many people have experienced this, to a milder extent, right before giving a public speech, performing in a concert, and so on. Treating the anxiety then, will reverse the problem.

Treatment: For the cold type: Follow the recommendations under treatment for cold hands and feet, emphasizing warming foods, spices and substances. Emphasize plenty of warm cooked meals and warm cooking styles such as soups, stews, baked casseroles, and hot drinks. Include more foods with heating properties in your diet according to body type: carrots, beets, onions, mushrooms, bell peppers, tomatoes, radish, artichokes, corn, olives, green grapes, plums, peaches, apricots, pineapple, oranges, mangoes, bananas, cranberries, cherries, cantaloupe, brown rice, oatmeal, granola, millet, corn tortillas, cornbread, chocolate, beef, poultry, seafood, pork, peanut butter/peanuts, walnuts, almonds, cashews, yogurt, cheese, eggs and lentils. Mulled apple cider, hot chocolate, warm milk with cinnamon, coffee, or any spicy tea with ginger or cinnamon are good hot drinks. Cut back the amount of sugar, soda, raw salads, tofu/soy products, and ice cream in your diet, as these foods are all cooling.

Kapha and kapha-pitta people can try simply garlic as a supplement or a ginger spicy tea internally to help warm the body. Vata and vata-pitta people can try ashwagandha or the Chinese formula rehmannia 8 taken internally to help warm the bladder and kidneys. Basically, any warming herbal formula will help stop this condition if it is due to cold. Vatas, vata-pittas, pitta-vatas, and pittas can also look at the advice under edema if they have it. The diet and herbal program should be somewhat warming for quite some time. Do your best to stay warm by dressing warm, and staying in well heated rooms and cars. Exercise can temporarily heat the body up somewhat, but for lasting warmth, warming foods, spices, and herbs are necessary!

For overactive bladder due to anxiety, work on releasing stress and fear.

27) Gas/Abdominal Bloating

Cause: In Chinese medicine, digestive problems are seen as a problem of the spleen, stomach or liver. In Ayurveda, each human being has a different set of laws governing his/her digestive tract. Certain foods and even natural substances will cause gas, colic, and bloating, depending on his or her body type. Those foodstuffs and combinations will repeatedly throw off digestion in that individual. In short, what one person can digest well, may cause bloating and gas in another person. For the vata type, aggravating foods will likely be dry, hard crunchy ones such as pretzels, cornbread, corn chips, popcorn, granola, barley, buckwheat, rye bread, broccoli, cauliflower, cabbage, Brussels sprouts, kale, collards, peas, legumes/beans, and dried fruits. For the pitta person, sour or fermented foods, and even spicy foods will cause bloating, gas, and diarrhea such as yogurt, sour cream, beer, wine, coffee, acidophilus, soy sauce, lemons, limes, barley malt, tempeh, grapefruit, sour fruits, sour juices, and too much chili powder. Kapha people will feel bloated after eating pasta, oatmeal, heavy starches, dairy foods, or sweets, as well as sour foods and fermented foods. Pitta-vata people will be aggravated by some vata aggravating foods and some pitta aggravating foods. The key to reversing this condition, is to avoid the foods which aggravate you and by following a diet that is right for your body system; the foods you were meant to digest well to begin with.

Treatment: **The vata person can take carminatives** (herbs that dispel gas) with meals such as hingwastak, cumin, coriander, sea salt, and asafoetida; or a mixture of ajwain, cumin, coriander, and fennel. Cardamom, cinnamon, ginger, and basil are also carminatives for this dosha. These spices/herbs can be taken as is or with some honey as a paste dissolved in the mouth with meals. Triphala, or just amalaki are good Indian herbs to help regulate digestion and prevent constipation in the vata digestive tract, as well as eating vata reducing foods such as sweet, sour, salty, or fermented items. They might also try a few pickles with each meal or a bit of wine, or umeboshi plum with dinner to improve digestion. Buttermilk is excellent. Vinegar and lemon juice in sauces are helpful as well as plenty of spices in your cooking. For natural supplements try betaine HCL tablets for insufficient acid in the digestive tract, and papaya enzymes taken with meals. Other digestive enzyme tablets are helpful. Do not use them if you have an ulcer, or heartburn. Some other herbs which strengthen the spleen in a vata predominant person are: licorice, ginseng, rehmannia, astragalus, ho-shou-wu, Solomon's seal, codonopsis, shatavari, amalaki, hawthorn berries, cinnamon, cardamom, ginger, orange peel, and sausserea. Look for formulas that contain a mixture of these herbs. The spicier herbs help counteract gas, bloating and nausea, while the heavier tonic starchy herbs like licorice, codonopsis, etc., help with constipation, dryness, and poor pancreatic function.

Vata-pitta people will have bloating and gas from both dry, crunchy hard foods and overly sour and fermented foods. Avoiding these both extremes, is helpful. In this case, a mixture of cardamom, fennel, and coriander is good taken with honey with meals. They too, can use the same spleen/stomach tonics, provided there is no nausea or diarrhea.

Pitta people will decrease intestinal discomfort if they avoid spicy, sour and fermented foods. Carminatives for them would be equal parts of fennel, cumin, cardamom, and coriander such as 1/4 teaspoon with meals or hot water poured over 1/2 teaspoon of this mixture drunk with meals. 7-10 drops of bitter gentian root extract with meals will help, since bitters help stimulate healthy liver and digestive function in these people. A Chinese condition called "liver invading the spleen" can cause the abdomen, over the liver area, to be chronically tender and bloated in these types. Symptoms of this condition are digestive disturbances such as bloating/gas, possible diarrhea, tenderness under the rib cage over the liver area, chronic headaches, breast soreness at the onset of the menses in women, an irregular menstrual period, irritability, feeling frustrated or angry often, and muscle neck, shoulder, or jaw tension. In this case, the focus in treatment should be the liver. Other liver regulating herbs for the pitta person are: milk thistle, bhumy amalaki, peony, bupleurum, dandelion, gardenia, turmeric, aloe vera gel, guduchi, burdock root, red clover, and grain coffees and teas made with chicory.

Kapha people can improve their digestion by including more bitters and pungent hot spices and foods in their diet as well as taking herbs with these properties. Dandelion, aloe vera, burdock root, turmeric, or bhumy amalaki are good bitters. Some pungent spices are: garlic, ginger, haritaki, pippali, clove, cinnamon, cardamom, and trikatu. The bitters can be combined with the pungent herbs for a good kapha digestive formula. If you are kapha-pitta predominant, the pungent warming herbs should definitely be mixed with something milder and cooler such as the bitters or cooling carminative spices. Some possible formulas, depending on the case are: cumin, coriander, and trikatu; ginger, punarnava, and aloe vera gel; or ginger, turmeric, coriander, and haritaki. A good Chinese herb formula for the kapha predominant person could include: saussurea, peony, atractylodes, poria, mint, magnolia bark, dandelion, and ginger, as this formula is drying and somewhat pungent.

28) Gingivitis

Cause: It is often believed among dentists that food particles become lodged in the spaces between the teeth and around the gums causing bacteria to proliferate leading to gum infection. Although this is true, especially if a person has poor hygiene and a build up of tartar, it is not always the case. Chronic inflammation of the gum tissue can also be caused from high pitta in the system. In other words, it is due to a diet that is too high in foods and substances that promote acidity, heat, and infection in sensitive individuals.

Treatment: Avoid pitta aggravating foods: mainly sour, spicy and acidic foods such as lemons, limes, papaya, grapefruit, yogurt, sour cream, buttermilk, pickles, cranberries, sour berries, green apples, bananas, kiwis, tangerines, tomatoes, coffee, alcohol, and vitamin C. Make a paste of turmeric and licorice, or neem and licorice with honey. Smear it on the gums everyday and leave on for several minutes. Turmeric and neem are natural antibiotics that will help fight infection topically. Internally, try a combination of shatavari, bala, or licorice root along with echinacea, neem, golden seal, bhumy amalaki, or turmeric if you are a vata or vata-pitta type individual. If you are kapha or kapha-pitta predominant, try any of the following natural anti-biotic herbs: echinacea, golden seal, bhumy amalaki, neem, gentian root, guduchi, or turmeric.

29) Hair Loss (in women)

Cause and Treatment: If a person is very young, sometimes the hair falls out due to clogged pores and follicles. In this case, a low fat diet or more kapha reducing foods will help. Circulatory promoting herbs such as ginger, garlic, and rosemary may be of help. A second cause occurs when an individual has a heat pattern in the body, causing the hair's roots to literally "burn" and break off. Heat dries up fluids and can dry out the scalp causing hair loss. In this case, decreasing heat in the body will reverse the problem. In 9 out of 10 cases however, hair loss is mainly caused from the scalp and hair becoming too dry with a deficient condition in the body developing (a high vata condition). Think of a tree when its leaves begin to change color and fall off in the fall season. The leaves change color and fall off as the tree becomes drier and chlorophyll production stops. Human hair doesn't change colors like a tree, but becomes drier as we age and when vata becomes elevated in the body. If there is much flaking on your scalp, dandruff, and your hair ends and texture feel dry or brittle, then I suspect it is falling out because you are too internally dried up, or "yin deficient." Some other symptoms of dryness are: dry lips, dry skin, dry nostrils, dry mouth, constipation, cracking in your joints.

No type of shampoo will completely reverse this, because the condition is an internal one like acne. Some shampoos, however, are worse than others for this condition. If the shampoo says it treats dry hair but contains chamomile, aloe, or rosemary, that isn't true. These herbs are all drying to the body internally and externally. What you want is a diet that is more moistening and a shampoo that has coconut oil, almonds, wheat, and/or citrus in it (fatty and sweet juicy substances). Also, do not wash the hair everyday. This just strips it of its natural oils. Moistening herbs for the hair are: ho-shou-wu, rehmannia root, Solomon's seal, bala, shatavari, licorice root, fennel, vamsha rochana, marshmallow, amalaki, triphala, and hawthorn berries. Even supplementing with vitamin C, A, and vitamin E are excellent for the hair because their sour and/or oily properties which help the body retain moisture. Flaxseed oil is another good supplement to try. Plenty of sweet fruit juices, bananas, kiwis, lemonade, oranges, pineapple, coconut milk, dates, fresh figs, red grapes, plums, melons, avocado, sweet winter squashes, pickles, cucumbers, pumpkin, brown rice, oatmeal, vinegar, yogurt, sour cream, tomato sauce, and ketchup are excellent moistening foods for strengthening and softening dry weakened hair. Follow a vata reducing diet, or emphasize more vata foods in your diet to reverse this condition. If you want to apply something natural topically, rub in olive, coconut, sesame, or almond oil into your scalp every night and rinse in the morning.

30) Heart Disease (high cholesterol-arteriosclerosis type)

Cause: The Western medical field strongly believes that elevated cholesterol in the body (especially high LDL and tryglycerides), along with high homocysteine and CRP (C-reactive protein) levels, increase the odds of a heart attack, as the arterial walls thicken and narrow due to fatty plague build up, and inflammation. Western medical recommendations for favorable cholesterol levels are: total count - under 200; HDL (good cholesterol) – above 60; LDL (bad cholesterol) - under 130; triglycerides (bad fats) - below 150; and a total lipid ratio under 4:1, or under 3:0 is ideal.

Although dietary cholesterol, when consumed in excess, can somewhat increase a person's lipid profile, I strongly believe genetics - an individual's body type, is the single greatest and strongest factor for elevated cholesterol levels in the human body. In Ayurvedic medicine, it is the pitta predominant person, or the person with a severe pitta imbalance, who falls into this category and is at greatest risk. Why is this so? For starters, pitta predominant people have a biological/genetic tendency towards what is referred to in Chinese medicine as liver congestion. Interestingly, in Western medicine, people with this genetic inheritance are also seen as people with a liver defect or lipid processing genetic defect. Both Western and Ayurvedic medicine believe the same thing. However, Ayurvedic medicine believes that dietary factors severely aggravate this genetic tendency turning it into a serious lipid metabolism problem.

Cholesterol basically comes from two main sources: all animal foods, and our own livers. The human liver makes its own cholesterol daily. When people, with genetically high cholesterol remove all sources of dietary cholesterol from their diets and their cholesterol still remains elevated, the source is their own liver. What then causes the liver to act faulty in this way? In Ayurvedic medicine, foods and substances that are both sour and fermented severely block up and create a congested liver in pitta predominant/genetic people. Hence, these type of foods are labeled pitta aggravating or pitta increasing, and they are far more deadly for raising cholesterol in the body than animal fats. They include: tomatoes, lemons, limes, grapefruit, papaya, strawberries, raspberries, blackberries, cranberries, kiwis, tangerines, rhubarb, granny smith apples, and basically any fruit that is sour or unripe that should otherwise be sweet. So while red delicious apples red grapes, and Bosc pears are considered sweet fruits, if they are eaten when sour, under-ripe, and frequent enough, they can pose a serious problem. Sour fruit juices are also extremely aggravating to liver function. Fermented substances are considered sour too, so they can cause the problem such as coffee, alcohol, yogurt, sour cream, buttermilk, cheese, pickles, miso, soy sauce, tempeh, sourdough bread, vegetarian mock meats, rice syrup, and barley malt. One of the biggest lies about vegetarianism, in my opinion, is that automatically adhering to such a diet devoid of animal food will automatically lower the cholesterol in these type of people or is the sole cause of their high cholesterol. Many soy or veggie alternative meats with labels spout “no cholesterol," but don’t tell you that they contain fermented sour substances such as soy sauce, nutritional yeast, and malt. The people with the greatest genetic sensitivity to sour and fermented foods will find that these specialty type foods give them severe gas and bloating in their abdomen when eaten, as do sour fruits and sour juices. However, other tests to check for pitta disturbances and makeup should be done.

Treatment: First, strictly avoid all sour, fermented and spicy foods and substances including vitamin C and acid products. If the fresh fruit in the supermarkets aren’t ripe enough or sweet, demand better quality produce and in the meantime, purchase canned fruits in syrup and add sugar to your fruit juices.

Second, consume more of these pitta reducing/liver friendly foods and make them the mainstay of your diet: kale, collards, lettuce, spinach, sprouts, avocado, green beans, peas, okra, artichokes, broccoli, asparagus, zucchini, sweet winter squashes, sweet potatoes, white potatoes, white sugar, mints, sweet red apples, sweet pears, sweet red grapes, prunes, sweet cherries, sweetened blueberries, sweet peaches, apricots, mangoes, melons, dates, figs, coconut, sweetened pineapple, sweet oranges, bananas with brown spots, and raisins. Watch the peaches, bananas, oranges and pineapple, as they tend to be more sour than sweet. In fact, even though they are listed here, if eaten exclusively only, they can still block up liver function. Also emphasize sweet types of dairy such as ice cream, milk, pudding, and ricotta cheese. Tofu is good, and for those people that can digest beans, they are also good. Whole grains to emphasize are whole wheat products, oat products such as oatmeal and oat based cereals, and rice.

Third, try herbs which help promote healthy liver function such as bitters: gentian, neem, dandelion, chicory, golden seal, turmeric, aloe vera, milk thistle, yellow dock, chlorophyll, bhumy amalaki, guduchi, and bupleureum. (Caution: If you are already taking prescription drugs or aspirin that is blood thinning, consult a practitioner before taking bitter herbs as this combination is not recommended.) Also, strictly avoid herbal recommendations for garlic and guggul, as these somewhat spicy or pungent herbs do not treat liver function, or help people with this genetic predisposition towards high cholesterol.

Fourth, minimize the amount and type of animal food you consume somewhat, as these foods when decreased, may lower cholesterol in the body slightly. The total amount of cholesterol in the blood, when decreasing these types of foods, will depend on genetics again. However, Americans as a group, tend to overindulge in their meat/animal food consumption, eating it three times a day in some cases. Often, many people will eat the worst forms too, such as fatty pepperoni, sausage, lunch meats, and whole milk. By the way, just for the record, poultry has the same amount of cholesterol as a 3oz. piece of lean beef. Chicken contains roughly 70 mg for the same 3-oz piece; fish still contains cholesterol - about 30 mg per 3-oz fillet on average. Eggs contain anywhere from 200 to 300 mg. A "lean" shoulder cut of pork has about 100 mg of cholesterol.

Last, quit smoking. Smoking constricts blood vessels, making the flow of blood through them difficult. Also watch out if you are taking birth control pills as they can also constrict blood vessels and arterial walls. In addition, be sure to participate in some form of exercise regularly to increase your HDL "good" cholesterol. Gradually work your way up. Consult a physician if you have any health problems before beginning any exercise program. However, do keep in mind that liver function has a greater impact on HDL levels than exercise. Decrease stress at work and home and/or find good coping skills to use or divert yourself from it.

31) Heartburn, Hyperacidity, Acid Reflux

Cause: Chronic heartburn, hyperacidity in the gut, or "acid reflux" as it is popularly named today, is caused from too much acidic, sour, fermented, and spicy foods which all increase acidity. This is a high pitta condition. Some people's bodies naturally tend to produce more hydrochloric acid genetically, and therefore should avoid an acid diet. To stop heartburn, avoid foods with these properties such as: tomatoes, lemons, limes, kiwis, bananas (especially when on the green side), papaya, rhubarb, sour berries, strawberries, cranberries, green apples, grapefruit, any fruit that happens to be sour or under ripe, yogurt (especially plain unsweetened), sour cream, buttermilk, sourdough breads, miso, too much orange juice or even sour pineapples. Any fruit or juice that is sour will aggravate this medical condition. When choosing fruit, pick ripe, very sweet tasting ones, or fruits in a sugary type syrup/juice. This is the one exception when canned fruit may be a better alternative to the natural unprocessed varieties. Also, avoid chili powder, chilies, horseradish, curry, garam masala, hot sauces, too much garlic, black pepper, cloves, ginger, cinnamon, mustard, ketchup, vinegar, gourmet and vinaigrette salad dressings, pickles, olives, alcohol, coffee, vitamin C, betaine HCL, and digestive enzyme tablets.

Treatment: For vata, vata-pitta, and pitta predominant people - try slippery elm, shatavari or licorice root powder mixed with honey (1/4-1/2 tsp.) with meals. These herbs can be also be taken in capsules. The bitter Indian herb neem or western bitter herbs golden seal, or gentian can be added to make the herb formula even stronger. All bitter herbs are anti-acids. Since most vata type people are sensitive to them, they should always be combined with heavier moistening herbs like the ones mentioned above. Milk, vanilla ice cream, vanilla pudding, white rice, white potatoes, white sugar, purple grapes, coconut, melons, red apples, pears, dates, figs, winter squashes, broccoli, cucumbers, and asparagus are great anti-acid foods. Even soda can help stop acidity in the gut, as sugar neutralizes acid.

You may also try 1/4 tsp. of cumin, fennel and coriander mixed together in equal parts.

If you are a kapha, kapha-pitta person, and have no nausea associated with the heartburn, try peppermint, chamomile, mullein, red raspberry leaf or dandelion tea (2- 3 cups day). Dandelion root, gentian root, neem, bhumy amalaki, red clover, turmeric, and even golden seal capsules, taken with meals, are stronger. Follow a kapha, or kapha-pitta diet while emphasizing kale, collards, white potatoes, broccoli, cauliflower, plain cabbage, peas, asparagus, green beans, sweet red apples, and sweet pears.

32) Heavy Menstrual Bleeding, Prolonged Bleeding, or Spotting between Periods (menorrhagia)

Cause: If fibroids, cysts, cancer, or a benign tumor is ruled out, heavy bleeding in the body is usually caused from too much dampness and heaviness in the system from eating too many heavy, watery, rich foods which increase blood volume and density. Kapha, kapha-pitta, and pitta type women are most prone to this, although any woman can have this as a problem. Dairy products, especially yogurt, winter squashes, sweet potatoes, zucchini, cucumbers, tomatoes, grapefruit, lemonade, kiwis, pineapple, oranges, bananas, melons, coconut, grapes, oatmeal, rice, fruit juices, and tofu are heavy, moist foods and will definitely promote the production and increase of blood volume in the body, including menstrual blood.

Spotting between the periods, simply means a heat imbalance is present in the body. Heat can cause blood to move quicker, overflow, or leak into the different channels of the body. Heat can cause breakthrough bleeding. Damp heat can make the blood flow quite heavy, as well as making the menstrual period last beyond the normal five days.

Treatment: A few weeks or months of the Indian herbs manjistha, arjuna, musta, ashoka, or the Western herbs nettle, dandelion, uva ursi, and plantain can help dry up blood volume. Also, try drinking 1-2 cups of red raspberry leaf, mullein, agrimony, and peppermint tea a day for three to 6 weeks. Neem and goldenseal are cooling herbs which can stop heat in the body causing spotting or lengthened bleeding. For heat, be sure also to follow a cooling diet (see the section under hot flashes). Avoid those foods which aggravate pitta. Avoid hot or strong spices, garlic, black pepper, cinnamon, too many warming and fermented foods. If you have bloody stools, see a medical doctor for an evaluation to rule out any other potentially serious problems. Beware that the above listed herbs are very drying as well as blood thinning, and can cause constipation, dryness of the mouth, sinuses, and nipples in some cases.

If the blood volume is heavy, avoid too many heavy watery foods such as too many sour or sweet foods like ice cream, yams, lemonade, zucchini, tomatoes, grapefruit, kiwis, oatmeal, bananas, winter squash, pumpkin pie, tomatoes, yogurt, sour cream, ice cream, alcohol, pickles, olives, oranges, and pineapple.

If there is anemia associated with your bleeding due to the hemorrhaging, consult a physician as well. Iron tablets, black strap molasses, and iron containing foods such as spinach, beets, and beef are helpful. Yellow dock contains iron and may be helpful for the kapha individual. However, remember that in this particular case, the root cause of the anemia is excessive bleeding which must be stopped to reverse the anemia. Read the section under anemia in this book for other suggestions.

33) High Blood Pressure (hypertension)

Cause: There are many causes for this serious medical problem. In some cases, excess water or edema in the body can drive blood pressure up in certain individuals. This is called a kapha type of high blood pressure. Heavy, watery foods will aggravate and contribute to this type. Also, heart disease/high cholesterol can cause high blood pressure, making the heart work harder to pump blood through narrow, clogged or constricted arteries. In pitta, pitta-vata, vata-pitta, and kapha-pitta predominant people, high blood pressure can be a complication of elevated heat and constriction in the body. As heat rises in the human body, it expands causing arterial pressure. Excessive heat in the body comes from both genetic factors (lots of pitta in the body) and too many heating foods such as: a high meat diet, nuts, brown rice, excess salt, alcohol, coffee, yogurt, cheese, tomatoes, carrots, beets, peppers, oranges, pineapple, bananas, peaches, miso, soy sauce, excessive garlic, ginger, cinnamon bark, curries, spicy foods. Any heating type herb will exacerbate hypertension, including ginseng, garlic, ginger, hawthorne, etc. In Chinese medicine, this type of hypertension is called the "yang type." Anybody can develop high blood pressure simply from eating too many animal foods, sodium, and not enough cooling fruits, leafy greens, milk, ice cream, or sweet fruit juices and sugars (White sugar and milk help lower high blood pressure!) Meat is also higher in sodium than fruits and vegetables. Produce tends to contain more potassium and sugars. Throwing off this ratio can also drive up blood pressure. Vegetarians as a group, on average, have fewer problems with high blood pressure than meat eaters.

General Advice For Everyone: My first suggestion, is to cut back meat consumption, avoid spicy foods, alcohol, and coffee, as well as consume less fat in your diet, and include more fruits and vegetables. Center your meals around produce, and plenty of salads, instead of meat as the main dish. Do not neglect milk and ice cream or sweet red grape juices as they can help lower blood pressure.

For the kapha, kapha-pitta type of high blood pressure, follow a kapha-pitta reducing diet given in the beginning of this book. There will be much weight, heat, and fluid retention in the body. Reduce fatty foods, spicy foods, as well as heavy, wet foods like bananas, kiwis, lemonade, oranges, pineapple, papaya, yogurt, sour cream, cheese, cottage cheese, ricotta cheese, nuts, oatmeal, lunch meats, sausage, pepperoni. Consume plenty of kale, collards, salads, asparagus, peas, green beans, apples. For fats, cholesterol, and heat in the blood stream, use bitter herbs such as neem, gentian root, or golden seal. Try including a tea brewed from skullcap, hops, and catnip to relax the nerves. For the fluid retention, try the cooling herbal diuretic uva ursi. Do not stay on these natural diuretics for too long and exercise caution when taking them.

In pitta, pitta-vata type high blood pressure, there may also be anger, irritability, frustration, possible headaches, redness in the face, red tongue, feeling heat in the body, dark urine, rapid pulse, muscle and shoulder tension, or hot flashes in women. In this case, use cooling nervine herbs to calm heated emotions (such as brahmi and jatamansi: 1/4 teaspoon equal parts 2 times a day, or brew 1 cup of skullcap/catnip/peppermint tea -1 teaspoon herb mixture per cup of hot water, strain and drink sweetened if like). Either of these should relax an agitated system. Also try other bitters to bring heat and blood pressure down such as: neem, bhumy amalaki, golden seal, or gentian root (2 capsules 2-3 times/day). Aloe vera gel is another good bitter, and can be taken in quantities ranging from 1/8 to 1/4 cup twice a day, also. Do not take bitter herbs if you are already on blood thinning type medication, including aspirin. If there is also dryness in the body, add in herbs such as bala, shatavari, licorice, fo-ti, Solomon's seal, or slippery elm. (One word about licorice: licorice root, when combined with bitters, lowers this yang type hypertension in pitta and vata types. However, it will raise blood pressure in the kapha types who already have water retention, as licorice draws water into the tissues.)

Decrease the amount of meat and salt consumed. Avoid hot spices, garlic, black pepper, chili powder, salsa, cheese, yogurt, sour cream, pickles, alcohol, coffee, tomatoes, too much orange juice. Eat more sweet fruits and juices (red apples, pears, dates, figs, coconut, purple grapes, watermelon), and emphasize lots of green salads, steamed greens like kale, collards, and spinach, as well as potatoes, broccoli, avocado, asparagus, cabbage, okra, and peas. Center your meals around abundant produce, with an emphasis on pitta reducing foods. Lifestyle measures to take include walks and strolls in the coolness of the morning or evening, swimming in cool water, avoiding heat and the sun, inhaling aromas of vetiver, lavender, honeysuckle, vanilla, jasmine or gardenia. These help calm an irritated, angry pitta mind. Learn how to release anger and resentment in constructive ways such as therapy, yelling in the woods, punching a pillow, burning paper, etc.

34) Hot Flashes

Cause: Hot flashes are basically caused from too much heat in the body. Literally cooling the body down internally, eliminates them. Ayurvedic medicine refers to them as a pitta disorder. Other symptoms of heat in the body that may or may not be present are: a red face complexion, general heat intolerance, dark, scanty, yellow urine, a red tongue, excessive thirst, high appetite, and a rapid pulse.

Treatment: Basically any substance that is "cooling" will reverse and stop them. Teas composed of peppermint, lavender flowers, chamomile, dandelion, chrysanthemum, and/or red clover may help. For stronger action try herbal capsules or formulas with neem, gentian root, dandelion root, gardenia, peppermint, echinacea, isatis root, scuttellaris, or golden seal. (If you are vata predominant, combine the bitter herbs listed above with heavier, moist, mildly cooling herbs such as marshmallow, shatavari,

Solomon's seal, bala, kapikacchu, or licorice root). There are many excellent Chinese herbal formulas for clearing heat, or “purging fire," as they are often called. The buzz about soy and tofu in the diet for hot flashes is due to the fact that they have a cooling effect on the body. However, soy products are not the best choice for the kapha women, as their properties are heavy and damp and they promote water retention, weight gain and congestion in the body.

Other suggestions for cooling the body down: add a cool rinse to your showers or better yet, go for a swim frequently in cool water. Wear white, blue, or green colored clothing, stay in the shade and out of the sun, hide out in air conditioning environments, use coconut oil on the skin, and center your diet around cooling foods such as salads, steamed kale, collard greens, spinach, endive, lettuce, chicory, broccoli, peas, asparagus, cucumbers, zucchini, cauliflower, cabbage, green beans, red apples, pears, purple grapes, dates, figs, watermelon, honeydew, blueberries, coconut, soy or cow’s milk, vanilla ice cream, pudding, wheat products, white rice, white sugar, tofu, ricotta and cottage cheese, egg whites instead of yolks, white and sweet potatoes, and winter squashes. Think green! Cook with butter, margarine, soybean oil, sunflower oil, or canola oil, instead of the heating olive oil. Avoid hot spices or too many spices such as garlic, black pepper, chili powder, cinnamon, and ginger, as well as alcohol, coffee, bananas, peaches, apricots, cantaloupe, cranberry juice, tomatoes, papaya, carrots, radishes, yogurt, cheese, sour cream, miso, soy sauce, nuts, and too much animal meat. Also, take note of this: animal food, except for the suggested dairy above, is heating in its energy, hence one reason why people of northern climates crave it in the winter. Vegetarians as a whole, may find themselves colder more often than their meat eating buddies. To compensate for this, they can follow the recommendations under cold hands and feet, emphasizing those foods that naturally warm the body up.

35) Hypoglycemia (low blood sugar)

Cause: There are several causes for this medical condition. Some people believe hypoglycemia is the beginning stage of adult onset diabetes. The standard western explanation of hypoglycemia is this: the body produces too much insulin to lower a high blood sugar condition, but the sudden surge of insulin lowers the blood sugar levels too much, resulting in low blood sugar (hypoglycemia). People may not be eating enough complex carbohydrates such as whole grains and vegetables in their diet and consuming way too much candy, cake, soda, sugar, white flour products, coffee, and even too much natural fruit juice, which all cause a quick rise in blood sugar followed by a quick surge/drop. This effect can leave one feeling exhausted, hungry, dizzy, and shaky. Sugar and soda pop are monosaccarides, one molecule, or simple carbohydrates (simple sugars), which don't require much time to be broken down and absorbed into the blood stream for energy. Whole grains and vegetables help supply the body with even amounts of glucose/energy when broken down, because they are polysaccharides and take longer to be broken down, digested and absorbed into system. They give the body even amounts of energy, instead of quick up and down surges.

In Ayurveda, hypoglycemia can develop in anyone, but the treatment should be different, as the cause is different. For some individuals, the cause is a diet actually too low in "naturally" sweet foods, as well as complex carbohydrates. This is especially true in pitta and vata type people who have a greater biological need for naturally sweet foods. They seem to have weaker insulin sensitivity. I have seen low blood sugar restored to normal, verified by blood tests, when a pitta individual added naturally sweet foods back into her diet, including simple white sugars and sweet fruit juices such as grape and apple juice. For the kapha person, just the opposite is true. A diet void of naturally sweet foods, and higher in complex carbohydrates and vegetables, will help regulate healthy pancreatic function, as these types have greater insulin sensitivity.

Treatment: Vata and pitta people can emphasize these naturally sweet foods in the diet: purple grapes, red apples, pears, plums/prunes, cherries, apricots, peaches, melons, oranges, pineapple, coconut, dates, figs, bananas, mangoes, sweet winter squashes, yams/sweet potatoes, white potatoes, broccoli, salads, zucchini, okra, green beans, yellow summer squash, corn on cob, peas, asparagus, avocado, cucumbers, whole wheat products, oatmeal, sweet rices, milk, ice cream, and sweet fruit juices. Having a serving of a complex carbohydrate such as oatmeal, whole wheat cream of wheat, whole wheat pancakes, brown rice, whole wheat bread or pasta three times a day, will also help. They can take 2 capsules of an herbal formula containing mostly licorice root, shatavari, or slippery elm temporarily to help restore fatigue and normalize blood sugar. Gurmar is an excellent bitter Indian herb for regulating pancreas function, and can be added for this condition.

Kapha people need to watch too many sweet foods. Instead they should work on omitting desserts, bananas, grapes, coconut, dates, melons, pineapple, oranges, figs, winter squashes, oatmeal, too much wheat, dairy, yams, and zucchini. Their diet should emphasize more bitter, pungent and astringent foods such as those listed under the kapha diet section at the beginning of this book. Bitters, which will help regulate the pancreas and liver function, are: neem, golden seal, aloe vera gel, bhumy amalaki, dandelion, and turmeric.

36) Hypothyroidism (underactive thyroid)/ Hyperthyroidism (overactive thyroid)

Cause: The thyroid gland produces the hormone thyroxine, which controls the rate of chemical reactions in the body, including metabolism. According to Western medicine, the thyroid gland's production of thyroxine is contingent in part upon sufficient quantities of iodine in the diet. Disorders result when the production of thyroxine is either insufficient or excessive giving rise to hypothyroidism or hyperthyroidism. In natural medicine, foods contain either larger amounts of potassium or sodium naturally, as well as containing trace minerals, and specific energetic properties such as excessive moisture or dryness, affecting the thyroid gland, and body's metabolic activity. In kapha types, the thyroid becomes sluggish from too many heavy foods, water retention, lack of exercise, and excess weight, which all slow all the body's functions. In vata types, hypothyroidism develops due to general weakness and lack of strength in the body. This is especially the cause when there is much thinness or emaciation. Pitta types can develop either the vata or kapha type of hypothryroidism. Hyperthyroidism is seen as a vata disorder –overactivity of the thyroid and metabolism. This often results from too much dryness in the system and/or heat making the body's functions overactive. In Chinese medicine, hyperthyroidism is considered an excess yang disorder.

Treatment for hypothyroidism: Vata, Vata-pitta type people can use Irish moss or kelp for this condition. Seaweeds stimulate underactive thyroid function because they are high in iodine and minerals and more "yang." Yin, and other heavy herbs should also be included such as licorice root, Solomen's seal, or marshmallow root, as they help with weakness. Try 2 capsules 3 times a day. Sea salt is an excellent natural source of salt that contains iodine and should be used in cooking and as table salt. Some store brands of salt contain anti-caking substances and aluminum. Sea salt can be obtained from any natural grocery, and sufficient amounts of it should be added to the diet. How much? Salt to taste, so the foods taste flavorful, without tasting salty. You may also want to include seafood in your diet, as iodine is plentiful in it. The diet should be vata decreasing by containing plenty of heavy damp foods such as oatmeal, milk, icecream, tofu, yogurt, sweet fruit juices, winter squash, cucumbers, avocado, grapes, and bananas.

Kapha people can use neem, ginger, shilajit, punarnava, burdock root, dandelion, goldenseal, guggul, or guggul and trikatu with neem. For any water retention, try uva ursi as an herbal diuretic. A kapha reducing diet should be emphasized. Lots of regular vigorous exercise is also crucial to stimulating the body's metabolism and functions. In Chinese medicine, kapha reducing foods are more "yang" naturally, helping the body to become stimulated and more active.

Treatment for hyperthyroidism: As said earlier, this is a vata condition, as vata type individuals tend to suffer from overactive states such as hyperactivity, nervous anxiety, insomnia, heart palpitations, increased appetite, fast catabolic metabolism, rapid pulse, fast talking/speech, etc. This is due to vata's naturally fast nature in the body, which must be kept in check by foods and substances that slow vata dosha down.

The vata, vata-pitta, or pitta-vata person should emphasize heavy, watery foods in the diet such as more tropical and sweet juicy fruits and vegetables. Their qualities will help slow down the activity of the thyroid. Emphasize more: bananas, kiwis, lemonade, oranges, pineapple, coconut, red grapes, plums, peaches, apricots, dates, figs, melons, pears, avocado, mangoes, grapefruit, zucchini, tomatoes, artichokes, plantains, okra, winter squashes, sweet potatoes, pumpkin, oatmeal, wheat products, short grain rice, black cow's milk, ice cream, sweetened yogurt, cottage cheese, ricotta, peanut butter and jelly sandwiches, and tofu/soy products. Pitta types should avoid the sour fruits such as lemons, limes, papaya, grapefruit, and kiwis.

Herbs to help slow an overactive thyroid include: shatavari, licorice root, rehmannia root, Solomon's seal, slippery elm, ho-shou-wu, marshmallow root, vamsha rochana, or wild yam. Dosages can range from 2-3 capsules three times per day, depending on the individual's height and weight. Warm milk with poppy seeds, sugar, and 1/4 teaspoon of nutmeg, can also be used as a mild sedative at bedtime. Decrease aerobic activity. Take plenty of long soaks in the bathtub or swim in fresh water (up to 30 minutes at a time).

37) Impotence

Cause: The cause of this condition is often related to a deficiency in the body (high vata). A poor, nutritionally depleted diet, as well as too much exercise and physically demanding work can cause much of the body's "qi" (energy or vitality) to be spent up so that none is left for the bedroom. In other cases, poor or blocked up circulation can cause it, along with the progression of aging.

Treatment for the deficient vata type: To reverse impotency, try heavy tonification (strengthening substances that build up the body and counteract fatigue). Foods, supplements, and herbs should be extremely nutritive, heavy, and vata decreasing. The person should also get adequate rest by going to bed by 10 p.m. and waking up by 7:00 a.m. Excessive aerobic exercise should be avoided. The diet should include plenty of heavy nutritive type foods: dairy foods, rice, wheat, oatmeal, winter squashes, pumpkin, zucchini, yellow summer squash, artichokes, sweet potatoes, cucumbers, bananas, melons, grapes, apples, pears, cherries, apricots, peaches, kiwis, coconut, plums, dates, figs, mangoes, pineapple, oranges, lemons, limes, tomatoes, nuts, olives, chocolate, sweet juices, sugar, tofu, eggs, and seafood, poultry, and beef. Choose those foods that taste good to you above and emphasize them in your diet. Avoid too many draining foods such as: beans, leafy greens, cabbage, cauliflower, broccoli, Brussels sprouts, celery, peas, too many other legumes, millet, rye, buckwheat, amaranth, quinoa, cornmeal and masa products, cranberries, pomegranates and herbal teas such as chamomile, lemongrass, dandelion.

Include tonic herb formulas that include: ashwaganda, licorice, kapikacchu, shatavari, ho-shou-wu, amalaki, Solomon's seal, Siberian, Chinese or American ginseng. Avoid ashwaganda, amalaki, and ginseng in formulas if you are pitta predominant or have a history of headaches, migraines, irritability, anger, or high blood pressure.

Treatment for the overweight kapha type: follow a kapha or kapha-pitta reducing diet. get plenty of regular exercise. Avoid fatty, heavy, and watery type foods such as dairy products, citrus, tomatoes, bananas, and too much starch. Try any of the following herbs combined in formulas: neem, guggul, dandelion, ginger, golden seal, burdock root, garlic. For water retention, try uva ursi or cleavers.

38) Insomnia

Cause: Insomnia is more common in vata people, pitta type people, and thin people. Vata type people are especially susceptible to this since they tend to have weak nervous systems, suffer more often from nerve tissue deficiency, anxiety, and much lightness (air and ether) in their bodies, making them feel literally "ungrounded" and hyperactive. On the other hand, more and more people in society are developing this due to the increasing social and economic pressures placed on them. They go to bed with an "overactive" mind, and worried about everything. Generally, in my opinion there are two main causes for insomnia. One has to do with being "ungrounded," of light weight, and having an overactive mind, as I just said. The other has to do with an agitated liver. People with an agitated liver sometimes have one or more of these symptoms of liver congestion: chronic headaches, an irregular menstrual cycle, tenderness or pain over the liver area, soreness of the breast tissue right before the menstrual period, shoulder and neck muscle tension, diarrhea, a red flushed face, feeling irritated easily, frustrated or angry. In Chinese medicine, insomnia is sometimes caused from a disturbance of the heart "shen."

Treatment: For the ungrounded nervous type: emphasize a heavier vata reducing diet. Take in foods that are more nourishing, heavy, and conducive to building strong nerve tissue. These foods also make one feel more settled, confident, and grounded. Consume more wheat pasta, breads, oatmeal, rices, dairy foods, yogurt, ice cream, nuts, meats, tofu, grapes, oranges, pineapple, bananas, plums, kiwis, coconut milk, dates, mangoes, melons, figs, peaches, winter squashes, zucchini, yams, olives, okra, yellow summer squash, sweet fruit juices, tomato sauce, artichokes, pumpkin pie, seafood, beef. Try 2 capsules of the herbal sedatives jatamansi (an Indian herb) or valerian at bedtime with a glass of warm milk and a hefty pinch of nutmeg and sugar. Pure vata types can take 1-2 capsules of valerian at bedtime. Avoid valerian if you are pitta predominant or have migraines, chronic headaches, irritability, anger, hot flashes, inflammatory pain, or an irregular menstrual cycle. To build up nerve tissue, try over the course of a few months, formulas that contain some of these herbs: shatavari, ho-shou-wu, ashwaganda, ginseng, marshmallow, zizyphus seeds, ophiopogon, codonopsis, hawthorn berries, schisandra, amalaki, and licorice. They can be taken during the daytime. Avoid ashwagandha, ginseng, hawthorn, amalaki, and schisandra if you have irritability, anger, an irregular menstrual cycle, hot flashes, chronic headaches, inflammatory pain, or are a pitta predominant person. Most of the above herbs have a nice calming/settling effect on the heart shen as well.

The agitated liver type of insomnia is more common in pittas, pitta-kaphas, and kaphas. Avoid sour and fermented foods, along with strong hot spices (grapefruits, lemons, limes, papaya, kiwis, yogurt, sour cream, pickles, alcohol, coffee, tempeh, sourdough breads, rhubarb, strawberries, cranberries, tomatoes, curry, horseradish, chilies, etc.). Try drinking 1-2 cups of this tea before bedtime: equal parts of skullcap, hops, chamomile, lemon balm, and catnip, or you can try jatamansi as a sedative at night. During the day, try bitter, liver regulating herbs for a few weeks or find a formula that treats the liver. Aloe vera, bupleurum, golden seal, gentian root, burdock root, red clover, neem, bhumy amalaki, turmeric, or milk thistle are good.

39) Irregular Menstrual Cycle (35-60 days)

Causes: Some women lose their menstrual cycle altogether when their body fat drops too low from being overly athletic, anorexic, or from simply being too thin. Too much or too frequent exercise with low body weight, affect a woman's hormones by causing estrogen levels to drop. In this case, a woman needs heavy tonification and nourishing, moist foods to reverse this as well as a decrease in the quantity of athletic activity. Follow the suggestions under scanty menstrual periods. In macrobiotic terms she is too "yang." The absence of her period is a form of malnourishment in which she does not make enough blood. The Chinese call this condition blood and/or yin deficiency. In western medicine, this medical condition is called amenorrhea.

Women who have an irregular cycle that is due to neither of these causes and who are carrying a good amount of weight, usually have a condition known as "liver qi stagnation" in Chinese medicine. Western medicine believes that a late menstrual cycle is due to a lack of progesterone in the body. Interestingly, the liver plays a role in the release of hormones in a woman's body. The liver makes the hormone progesterone, and when there is a liver function problem, progesterone is not released and dispensed by the liver when it should be. In Ayurvedic medicine, this condition translates to a "pitta imbalance," which also means liver stagnation problem. Therefore, the condition will reverse itself by treating liver function such as: avoiding sour, spicy and fermented foods. Other red flag symptoms associated with this type of imbalance are: chronic headaches, possible migraines, yellowing under the arm pits, unjustified or exaggerated anger, irritability, frustration, loose stools or irritable bowel syndrome, heartburn, genetic high cholesterol, shoulder and neck muscle tension, and/or soreness over the liver area of the abdomen. A woman need not have every single one of these problems to have liver congestion.

A third reason for the lack of a menstrual period, may be cysts causing an obstruction of the flood of blood. An ultra sound is one test that may help detect this cause.

Treatment: For the first cause, consume more vata reducing foods and cut back on the exercise. Some herbs that build up blood volume include: ho-shou-wu, shatavari, licorice, rehmannia, jujube, Solomon's seal, and amalaki. Read the section in this book under scanty menstrual period/blood for more ideas. For anorexia, get into a treatment program that includes therapy.

For the second cause, use herbs and vitamins that regulate liver function: turmeric, aloe vera gel, milk thistle, bhumy amalaki, dandelion, neem, golden seal, red clover, burdock root, gentian root, chrysanthemum, and chicory grain coffee substitutes. The B vitamins are helpful to the liver as well. Avoid liver aggravating hot spices, bananas, kiwi, berries, papaya, plantains, rhubarb, strawberries, grapefruits, lemons, limes, green apples, green grapes, and cranberries. If any of these so called sweet fruits taste sour, they should be avoided or eaten in syrup or juice: plums, cherries, apricots, peaches, mangoes, oranges and pineapple. Fermented foods to avoid are: pickles, miso, soy sauce, tempeh, alcohol, coffee, yogurt, sour cream, sharp or hard cheeses, sourdough breads, and mock soy meats. Also avoid radishes, turnips, eggplant, beets, and too many tomatoes. A dish of greens (kale, collards, spinach, lettuce) 5 times a week initially, will help. The bitters in them stimulate healthy liver function. Have salads from spinach, romaine lettuce, green leaf, red leaf, Boston lettuce. Artichokes, asparagus and broccoli are also good food choices to emphasize in the diet. The bottom line is, pitta needs to be regulated.

40) Menstrual Cramps (dysmenorrhea)

Cause: There are many medical theories behind this disorder, such as a production of too many of the bad prostaglandins in the body. The common Western medical approach often involves putting the woman on hormone/birth control and pain relieving pills. Western holistic practitioners believe a lack of the minerals calcium and magnesium play a role in menstrual cramps, as these minerals help control muscle contractions. In Chinese medicine, the view is that it is caused from an obstruction of "qi." (An inharmonious movement of the vital energy of the sex organs, hormones, and energy flow in the lower abdomen area). The more blocked up that area becomes, the greater the chances of developing uterine cramps.

In my practice, I have found that this latter theory seems to be the most correct. I have personally found, with my patients, that women who have poor digestive function such as bloating and gas after meals, frequent constipation, loose stools, liver stagnation tendencies, or irritable bowel syndrome, are more likely to experience painful cramps than women who don't. I believe the key to reversing this disorder is to improve digestion, prevent or decrease liver congestion, and balance the doshas.

So, decide first what body type you are. Secondly, look for other clues to help you determine what is wrong. For example, if you have a tendency to be constipated and bloated frequently, chances are vata dosha is off balance causing the digestive disturbance and the cramps or spasms. If your tendency is to get headaches, diarrhea or loose stools, especially during your period, then it is most likely that pitta dosha is the cause of your problem. If you have a pattern of chronic headaches, muscle tension, an irregular menstrual cycle, sore achy breasts that come and go with your cycle, irritability, frustration, anger, and/or soreness below the right side of your rib cage over the liver area, it is most likely that liver congestion is playing some role in your menstrual cramps. Kapha people rarely get menstrual cramps, and in kapha-pitta people, the cause is almost always due to liver congestion or throwing pitta dosha off balance.

Treatment: For the vata type, follow a vata pacifying diet. Emphasize foods that are sour, mildly spiced, and oily to minimize gas, bloating and constipation. Avoid vata aggravating dry foods such as popcorn, beans, broccoli, cauliflower, cabbage, Brussels sprouts, peas, dried fruits, granola, corn grains. Try 2 capsules of triphala at nighttime with 1 glass of orange juice or purple grape juice if there is constipation. You may even want to try 1 cup of buttermilk or yogurt with 1/4 teaspoon nutmeg. During the day, try 1/4 teaspoon of hingwastak, coriander and cumin, or cumin, fennel, and cardamom with meals. Also add in 2 capsules 2x day of licorice root. While having cramps, take 1-2 capsules of valerian or 1-2 capsules (1/4-1/3 tsp.) of jatamansi. These are sedatives, pain relievers, and help with cramps. Do not take these sedatives/pain killers with aspirin or any other prescription drugs.

For a pitta imbalance – Avoid pitta aggravating foods such as sour, fermented and spicy foods. The stools should be normal and well formed. Include more pitta reducing foods in your diet. Try a mixture of equal parts of cumin, fennel, and coriander taken with meals to help dispel the gas. Also try 2-3 capsules a day of milk thistle, dandelion, turmeric, neem, bhumy amalaki, golden seal, or gentian root for a few weeks to regulate liver function. For a natural pain killer during your period, brew 1-2 cups of tea made from 1 teaspoon of these herbs mixed together (skullcap, hops, catnip, and peppermint). Strain and sweeten with sugar. You might also want to try 1-2 capsules of white willow bark or 1-2 capsules of jatamansi instead. Do not use the willow bark if allergic to aspirin.

For the pitta-kapha person – Eat foods for your body type/system/imbalance. Try drinking 1/8-1/4 cup aloe vera gel in the morning for several weeks prior to your next period. Also try 7-10 drops of gentian extract with your meals, and a combination of these spices: cumin, coriander, turmeric, and ajwain seeds, or ginger, cumin, and coriander to help regulate your digestion. For actual pain, try a tea made from skullcap, catnip, hops, and peppermint, and/or 1-2 capsules of either willow bark or jatamansi. Again, exercise caution, as these are sedatives. Some other Western and Chinese herbs for the kapha type to include in a formula for pain are: crampbark, bupleurum, angelica, dandelion, peony, thyme, lemon balm, and cyperus. If water retention is a consistent problem each month, be sure to eat more naturally drier and lighter kapha decreasing foods. You may want to use some herbal diuretics such as dandelion or uva ursi. If liver congestion is the problem, emphasize more pitta reducing type foods and use bitter herbs: neem, golden seal, dandelion, gentian root, or bhumy amalaki. Avoid sour, spicy, and fermented foods.

41) Migraine Headaches and Chronic Headaches

Cause: Headaches, including migraines, are completely reversible and preventable. A headache that comes on suddenly out of thin air and then vanishes and doesn't return for months at a time, is often caused by a pernicious external influence. For example, a person may develop a headache from running outside in the hot summer heat, or develop one from being exposed to drafty cold, or windy air. These are outside influences. Chronic, frequent headaches that happen day after day, or week after week, or every time right before the menstrual period like clockwork, are caused from an internal disharmony. In these cases, liver qi stagnation is the culprit. When the "qi" energy of the liver does not flow smoothly or in the proper direction, or its energy becomes stagnant, congested, a headache or migraine develops. Treat the liver and the headaches start to disappear.

Treatment: Basically this is a pitta condition, as pitta is responsible for liver congestion in the body. Following a pitta decreasing diet will help tremendously, since many pitta decreasing foods help regulate the liver's function. These foods include bitter greens, milk, ice cream, and sweet fruits such as red apples, pears, red grapes, dates and coconut. Avoid sour foods, fermented and spicy foods such as pickles, feta and sharp cheeses, lemons, limes, sour berries, cranberry juice, strawberries, grapefruit, papaya, kiwis, bananas, orange juice, yogurt, sour cream, alcohol, coffee, chilies, horseradish, curry powder, cloves, too much black pepper, too much garlic, cinnamon, raw onions, tomatoes, and any fruit that happens to taste sour or be unripe. You made need to add sugar to the so-called "sweet" fruit juices (like grape and apple juice) to decrease their sourness.

Try herbs that stimulate and regulate healthy liver function such as bhumy amalaki, neem, golden seal, dandelion root, turmeric, milk thistle, burdock root, red clover, yellow dock, feverfew, or bupleurum. In severe cases, try also drinking 1/8 –1/4 cup of aloe vera gel for three to four weeks as well. For pain while having a headache or migraine, try some natural pain relievers that also affect the liver: a tea composed of the following herbs: skullcap, catnip, hops, peppermint, and chrysanthemum, along with 1-2 capsules of white willow bark or jatamansi. Some of these herbs are sedatives as well as bitter, so do not combine them with over the counter or prescription pain killers and sedative drugs. Another good tea for liver related headaches, although not pain relieving, is chrysanthemum, feverfew, and peppermint tea. Do not take any of the herbs listed above if you are already on blood thinning prescription drugs. Also do not take large doses of vitamin E with bitter herbs. Vata and vata-pitta people should include a heavy herb formula to offset the effects of the drying bitters, such as formulas that include any of the following herbs: licorice root, shatavari, ho-shou-wu, rehmannia, marshmallow, Solomon's seal, or kapikacchu. Avoid these heavy herbs if nausea is present.

One last piece of advice: if you feel a migraine or headache just starting to come on, eat a salad with a sweet dressing, a dish of steamed kale or collard greens, a dish of vanilla ice cream, and/or have a soda. These will help open up the blocked liver energy. Avoid the ice cream and soda if nausea is also present.

42) Nausea/Lack of Appetite

Cause: Kapha in your system has become too high, regardless of your constitution (body type). Too much internal dampness, food stagnation, and/or possible cold are putting out your digestive fire, which is your appetite. Your diet is too full of heavy, sweet, rich, oily, sour, cooling and/or bland foods. Maybe you are eating too much food in quantity, or eating too often. Look to see if the tongue has a greasy, white, thick coating, if your saliva is thick, if you have loose stools, a loss of the sensation of taste of foods, or maybe recent weight gain, which are other signs of internal dampness. Lack of appetite can also be due to low pitta, a case where your digestive fire is low, but it does not necessarily mean high kapha. It means your diet is not acidic, warming, or spicy enough to keep your appetite "stoked." Think of your appetite as a campfire. The bigger the fire, the bigger the appetite. To stoke the fire, one needs plenty of dry, light wood, not heavy, damp, cold logs, especially if the fire is weak.

Treatment: Temporarily emphasize light, dry, warm, kapha decreasing, somewhat spicy, or well seasoned foods in your diet, depending on your tolerance for spicy foods. A few days of eating only light meals such as Mexican food, tacos, bean burritos, light soups, salads, chili, corn chips, popcorn, crackers, steamed greens, baked potatoes, onions, mushrooms, broccoli, salt, pepper, garlic, or chili powder, will help reverse this problem. Avoid heavy foods such as sweet fruit juices, pineapple, oranges, bananas, lemonade, milk, ice cream, yogurt, sour cream, desserts, peanut butter, too many starches, oatmeal, and anything sweet, or gooey. If spicy foods bother you, take mild spices like basil, cooked garlic, cinnamon, turmeric, black pepper, oregano, sage, etc. You might want to try a 1/8-1/4 teaspoon of a spice mixture with your meals to stimulate appetite: hingwastak and cumin; pippili, cumin, coriander and trikatu; dry ginger, black pepper, cumin and coriander. Simple ginger and cumin or black pepper and cumin will also do. There are some excellent Chinese herb formulas to decrease nausea which include herbs such as saussurea, magnolia bark, poria, atractylodes, pinellia, radish, citrus peel, ginger root, and bupleurum. Be careful with pinellia, as it is considered toxic. Spicy teas like ginger root tea, light cranberry juice, black tea, or plain black coffee can also help alleviate nausea. In mild cases, seltzer water can help, because the carbonation adds air back into your digestive track.

If your fire has simply been lowered, and you are also physically cold all the time, slowly add more warming as well as acidic foods into your diet. Vitamin C, digestive enzyme and HCL tablets, cranberry juice, orange juice/oranges, pineapple, tomato sauce dishes, ketchup, barbecue sauce, mustard, garlic, black pepper, chili powder, vinegar dressings, yogurt, pineapple, kiwis, papaya, and lemonade are good picks. Also read under the section for treating cold hands and feet in this book (part 6), for more ideas.

43) Oily and Damp Skin

Cause: Large, overweight kapha type or kapha-pitta type people usually have this condition. In cases of damp skin, the palms will feel moist or clammy. You may sweat very easily even without exercising, heavy exertion, or without being overheated. The skin will feel oily or there will be boils or blackheads on the face, back and neck. Humidity will probably bother you. You may even have edema, such as swelling around your ankles or puffy fingers. If this is the case, read the section under edema (part 6) in this book.

Treatment: For kapha internal dampness, eat a drier diet. Avoid damp foods like oatmeal, grapefruit, lemons, limes, melons, kiwis, bananas, yogurt, sour cream, too much dairy food, coconut, avocados, tomatoes and tomato sauce, nuts, winter squashes, sweet potatoes, globe artichokes, cucumbers, zucchini, olives, pickles, and seafood. For oily skin, avoid fatty foods such as fried foods, peanut butter, nuts, avocados, coconut, tahini, soy products, potato chips, cheese, fatty meats, hidden oils in baked goods, butter, etc. Follow food suggestions for the kapha or kapha-pitta type. For acne, follow the suggestions under acne in this book.

44) Osteoarthritis

Cause: Osteoarthritis is a deterioration of the cartilage matrix in the knees, hips, joints, and spine, and has several causes including exercising too frequently or strenuously, putting too much friction on the joints such as the knees, suffering from a serious injury, or an underlying deficiency/malnourishment condition (metabolic problem) in the body. What occurs in some cases, are tiny fractures that cause cartilage to break off. Cartilage also becomes weak, thin and frail as it becomes dried out from lack of blood, synovial fluid and other fluids in the joints. Collagen production is important, because it is one of the several factors influencing cartilage production.

In my opinion, the single greatest cause of osteoarthritis is a metabolic, deficiency problem. Cartilage is one of the main tissues in the human body like muscle, bone, fat, blood, plasma, etc. If the body remains in a deficiency or catabolic state continuously over a long period of time, the body's tissues suffer. Vata types, vata-pittas, and pitta-vatas are the most genetically prone to this disorder. Thin people, in general, tend to develop tissue deficiency problems more easily. A diet deficient in heavy, moistening, rich, nourishing tissue building foods is the other main culprit. Eating too many "air" foods like salads, broccoli, cauliflower, cabbage, Brussels sprouts, white potatoes, peas, kale, collards, beans/legumes, dried fruits, granola, corn chips, and popcorn can cause and exacerbate this. This person needs plenty of dairy products, meats, seafood, nuts, oatmeal, rice, wheat, fruit juices, pineapple, oranges, bananas, peaches, grapes, winter squashes, tomatoes, zucchini, etc., to reverse this disorder. (I have seen many young women in my office with the beginning stages of this disorder due to being on restrictive diets in the name of weight loss. Live on exclusively salads and beans, especially if you are a small woman, and your odds of developing this serious medical problem increase significantly.)

Treatment: Include many of these foods and substances in your diet: vinegar, vitamin C, pickles, cheese, sour cream, milk, ice cream, yogurt, oatmeal, rice, wheat bread, pasta, peanut butter, beef, poultry, seafood, olives, tomatoes, zucchini, winter squashes, yams, artichokes, avocado, cucumbers, grapes, plums, dates, apricots, peaches, melons, figs, coconut, pineapple, oranges, mangoes, lemonade, kiwis, papaya, grapefruit. Sour foods are high in vitamin C, which helps improve flexibility, build collagen in the body and help increase fluid in the body. Any of the following heavy herbs will help restore lubrication and strengthen cartilage as well as bone: bala, ho-shou-wu, Solomon's seal, licorice root, shatavari, wild yam, marsh-mallow, vamsha rochana, and rehmannia root. Hawthorn berries and amalaki are sour herbs that may also help some individuals. Although many herbal formulas contain anti-inflammatory herbs for pain, such as turmeric, willow bark, skullcap, dandelion, neem, aloe vera, or red clover, these herbs actually contribute to the destruction of cartilage. If you decide to use them, always be sure to combine them with at least twice as much of the heavier joint building herbs listed. Glucosamine sulfate, chrondroitin, and vitamin C are some other supplements thought to rebuild cartilage or help slow its progression. Make sure your diet contains plenty of naturally sweet, heavy, sour, moist, cartilage building foods, supplements and herbs.

45) Osteoporosis

Cause: Osteoporosis is often referred to as the silent, but potentially deadly disease. Although people in the medical profession claim that only bone scans/x-rays help detect it, I personally think that there are other warning symptoms. Some of these visible signs are: a humpback or hunch back curving of the spine, receding gums in the mouth since the gums shrink as the tooth shrinks (the tooth is bone material), and bone spurs on the feet or elsewhere. In my opinion, vata and pitta predominant men and women seem to be most biologically susceptible to this, because of their tendency to suffer from deficiency type diseases. Pitta women tend to be acidic and even too much acid can dissolve bone. However, osteoporosis is a disease that can affect anyone. It is true that our bodies store larger amounts of calcium and minerals when we are younger, and this process slows and halts as we age. Menopause affects women too, because as estrogen production decreases, its protection of bone loss decreases as well.

However, certain substances and foods can accelerate or make people more vulnerable to this serious condition. For starters, too much acidic foods in the diet, can cause calcium to be leached from the bones such as: vinegar, coffee, wine, alcohol, tomatoes, ketchup, pickles, olives, lemons, limes, kiwis, rhubarb, papaya, grapefruit, sour berries (strawberries, cranberries), green apples, sour plums, too many bananas, too much orange juice, or sour peaches. Sour cream, buttermilk, as well as too much yogurt, especially the plain, unsweetened kind, can also aggravate this condition. Anything that is fermented or sour has an acid forming effect on the human body. The more naturally acidic you tend to be, the more devastating these type foods will have on your body, including your skeleton. Also, a lack of calcium in the diet can contribute to this problem.

Treatment: Take calcium supplements with magnesium, vitamin D, and boron for the best absorption of the calcium. Shoot for a total consumption of 1500mg of calcium a day. Your supplement should have twice as much calcium as magnesium in it. Although other practitioners often recommend calcium citrate, as it is more easily absorbed and broken down in the body, some people's bodies are already very acidic and can break down calcium carbonate. Look for supplements in health food stores, because the quality of the products they get is usually superb. Avoid getting your calcium from dolomite, oyster shells, and anti-acid formulas advertising calcium. Many of these products contain aluminum, as well as lacking the needed mineral magnesium.

Alkalize your diet by eating more pitta reducing foods that are less acidic. Include more of these high calcium, acid buffering foods in your diet: kale, collard greens, carrots, broccoli, bok choy, Brussels sprouts, okra, green and red leaf lettuce, green beans, parsnips, sesame seeds or tahini, almonds, tofu and soy products, legumes, figs, raisins, prunes, milk, cottage cheese, cheese, ice cream, and seafood like scallops, lobster, or clams, sardines. Sweeter type fruits to eat more often are: red apples, pears, grapes (especially the red ones), raisins, dates, figs, prunes, sweetened cherries, dried apricots, cantaloupe and melons, coconut. Although dairy products are a potent source for calcium, they aren't the only source of calcium. One cup of steamed collard greens has 357 mg of calcium, 2 T of sesame seeds have 218 mg of calcium, 3 raw carrots have 90 mg of calcium, and 1 cup of broccoli has 132 mg, according to Laurel Robertson in her book: *The New Laurel's Kitchen.* Exercise helps increase bone density, and should be included in a prevention/treatment game plan. The more resistance or heavier the type of exercise, the better, such as weight lifting.

Vata type people should consume plenty of heavy foods and substances such as rice, wheat, oatmeal, winter squash, yams, artichokes, zucchini, cucumbers, milk, cheese, yogurt, cottage cheese, tofu, almonds, tahini, figs, and sardines for calcium sources.

46) Overweight/Obesity

Cause: This results from many different causes such as an underactive thyroid, eating to medicate one's emotions, compulsive overeating, eating too many calories in general, no exercise, high fat diets which tend to be calorie dense, repeated yo-yo diets, having a genetically slow metabolism (kapha body type), etc.

I strongly believe in the Ayurvedic view of body/genetic type differences between people, which results in different metabolic rates. This is why you can put several different people on the same calorie and exercise plan, and not all of them will lose weight or lose the same amount of weight. Also eating when one is not truly hungry, or eating to the point of feeling stuffed, is the single greatest cause of obesity besides body type/genetics. In this case, no healthy eating plan in the world can help someone lose weight if they are using food to medicate emotions such as anger, boredom, self pity, depression, anxiety. Professional counseling is an excellent choice, for this person.

Another common pitfall is the concept of "going on a diet," which sets up the individual to fail immediately, because it means following an eating plan that is impossible to keep up or live on for the rest of one's life. Deprivation of one's favorite foods, is likely to cause a dieter to fail. Also, self-sabotaging thought patterns prevent people from losing weight, such as when a person starts a new healthy regime and exercise plan, has several pieces of cake, ice cream, or other fatty foods, then thinks they "blew it," so they might as well give up. The better way to handle that type of situation is to compensate for the fatty or high calorie foods in one meal, by consuming lighter, healthier foods throughout the rest of the day or week, and not to skimp on the exercise. For example, suppose you ate pancakes, donuts, orange juice, or sausage and eggs for breakfast, and then later on in the day went for a walk and had fresh fruit, a salad, a baked potato, and beans. This way, the concept of "blowing it" doesn't exist.

The other traps people fall into, are high protein, low carbohydrate diets. They are so attractive to many people because weight loss seems "fast" in the first few weeks. However, what really occurs is water loss, not weight loss, as carbohydrates hold water in the body. High protein diets are also extremely dangerous because they increase one's likelihood of developing cancer, and in some cases, hypertension, not to mention putting a huge strain on the liver and kidneys since meats are diuretic, and contain many harmful nitrates and antibiotics. Yes, a certain reduction in the total amount of carbohydrates can help, but their total restriction is not necessary. Depriving oneself of all carbohydrates including the healthy complex carbohydrates, like brown rice, potatoes, pasta, and cereals, can cause blood sugar levels to plummet in some people. Sugar is one source of fuel/energy for the body, and all types of carbohydrates are eventually broken down into sugars. When total carbohydrate deprivation occurs, the body sends out messages to consume simple carbohydrates like candy, for immediate energy. This process sets the person up for a binge on sweets.

Pushing these factors aside, consuming more kapha reducing or lighter foods can help weight loss considerably, along with an exercise plan and reducing calories. Eating too many heavy foods, especially at each meal, will promote weight gain. For example consuming oatmeal, milk, and a banana or sausage and eggs for breakfast; non-fat yogurt for lunch or peanut butter and jelly; a candy bar as a snack; pizza or spaghetti with tomato sauce and meat-balls with cheese for dinner; and cream pie, ice cream, or cake for dessert will make weight loss more difficult. Having a roast beef or cheese sub or cheese burger, fries, and a milkshake or ice cream cone, is a high calorie meal. People eat this kind of regime, don't exercise, and wonder why they can't lose weight. They think they are cursed or something. Fatty foods are often more calorie dense, and calorie deficit still has to occur for weight loss, either through calorie reduction and/or exercise/activity. However, low fat diets are sometimes not helpful, since they are not as filling in the stomach and cause people to over-eat. Not everything that is lowfat is low in calories. You have to read labels.

Treatment: Try emphasizing more apples, pears, raisins, grapes, plums, prunes, cranberries, strawberries, raspberries, cherries, blueberries, peaches, apricots, pomegranate, persimmons, broccoli, cauliflower, cabbage, Brussels sprouts, kale, collards, spinach, Boston lettuce, green and red leaf lettuce, romaine, mustard greens, leeks, radishes, carrots, peas, green beans, yellow wax beans, all legumes except soy products, sprouts, celery, beets, turnips, rutabaga, burdock root, bok choy, bell peppers, potatoes, corn on cob, cornbread, popcorn, rye breads, millet, barley, quinoa, amaranth. Again, it is wise to avoid those foods suggested here that either taste unpleasant, cause bloating and gas, or are not satisfying to you. They may not be right for your body type. Use intuition. Try fruits for breakfast or cereal and skim milk; salad or stir fried vegetables over pasta, or soup w/crackers for lunch; and any combination of light foods for dinner. Breakfast might also be an egg omelet with onions and bell peppers. Lunch might be vegetarian chili and crackers with steamed kale, dinner could be a baked potato with broccoli, and steak. For dessert try fruit pie. Lighten up! If you are only a bit overweight and more of a medium sized vata-pitta or pitta person, eat more produce, less starch, less oily foods, and use lowfat dairy products and egg whites.

Also start an exercise program if you haven't already done so. Pick something you like and do it 4-5 times a week. Be consistent with it. An aerobic exercise program and weight lifting are the best combination for weight loss. Aerobics burn calories and speed up the metabolism, while weight lifting creates lean muscle tissue, which increases the metabolism by eating up more calories even while at rest. It takes more calories to maintain one pound of muscle than it does to maintain one pound of fat. Fat is inactive. Muscle will also make you look leaner, add shape to your body, and help reduce clothing size. When seeking to reduce weight, forget the scales and be more concerned with body fat percentage. Also, be leery of the image conveyed by models in magazines. Many of them have eating disorders or are drug users. Their image is not necessarily one of health.

47) Poor Memory

Cause: Many experts disagree as to the exact cause of this condition and degenerative memory diseases such as Alzheimer's. Some argue that genetic high cholesterol causes it. There is even speculation and research about countries that eat highly processed and fatty food diets and higher incidences of Alzheimer's disease. What is of most interest to me is that in some countries, the disease doesn't even exist. So is it about the United States lifestyle, diet, or environment that contributes to this disorder?

Scientific evidence exists showing the clumping and entanglement of nerve masses in the brains of Alzheimer's patients. According to an article in *Alternative Medicine* magazine, issue 25, by Richard Leviton called "Brain Power Repair for Alzheimer's;" brain cells die as they become entangled with protein deposits. Leviton also states that the hormone cortisol, produced mainly from stress and free radicals, contributes to the killing of brain cells. He says that other research points to the decline of acetylcholine in aging people; a chemical that helps play a role in memory. Another article, in *Time*, "(Our Daily Folate," May 24, 1999, pp. 72-73), cited a link between diets deficient in folate and memory impairment. This comes as no surprise to me, because it has been long known in alternative medicine, that the B vitamins play a role in the nervous system and vitamin B deficiencies can cause memory impairment. While what causes their uptake in the body to become impaired or prohibited is somewhat unknown, some studies have found that high concentrations of aluminum in the brain, and other toxic substances, may play a role. Furthermore, consuming a lifetime diet of white flour, white bread, white rice, refined starches void of B vitamins, and leafy green vegetables isn't helpful.

Treatment: Because the exact cause of memory impairment diseases like Alzheimer's is unknown, my suggestions are only based on hypotheses, may not work, but are as follows: 1) Avoid the intake of processed food as much as possible, while also consuming only whole grain products like brown rice and whole wheat breads, as these foods are also high in B vitamins. 2) Avoid aluminum cans, foil, baking dishes, foods, and products that contain it such as deodorants, and baking powder. Bake with Rumford baking powder instead. 3) Drink filtered water. 4) Consume plenty of leafy greens such as kale, collards, romaine lettuce, green leaf lettuce, Boston lettuce, spinach, and Brewer's yeast, legumes, or wheat germ. These foods are naturally high in B vitamins. 5) Include daily a super B-complex vitamin with lecithin in it. Pick a formula with 25 – 50 mg. 6) You might want to try herbs such as brahmi, shank pushpi, and ginko. These herbs have been known to increase mental awareness by improving blood flow to the brain and acting as free radical scavengers. In Ayurveda, they are considered mental stimulants. Peppermint, sage, basil, sassafras, and coffee also act as mild nervine stimulants. If you are taking any blood thinners, beware that ginko and brahmi have anti-clotting properties and might not be a good combination. 7) Co Q-10 is a natural anti oxidant supplement thought to help the body's cellular energy (ATP) production, and act as a free radical scavenger. It may also be useful in memory impairment. 8) If you are vata, vata-pitta, or pitta individual, sometimes a failing memory can be due to nerve deficiency in which case, tonic herbs that help build up nerve tissue are necessary. Try using a combination of some of the following nerve building herbs as part of a formula: ashwagandha, shatavari, licorice root, Solomon's seal, ginseng, vamsha rochana, wild yam, slippery elm, rehmannia, and ho-shou-wu. Avoid ginseng and ashwagandha if you are a pitta predominant person. Oily vitamins such as A, D, E, and C can be supplemented to the diet, along with B complex.

Last, another type of mental dysfunction can occur, especially in kapha predominate people. This type involves lethargy, grogginess, and lack of mental clarity. The person needs several hours in the morning to feel mentally "alert" after waking up. This lethargic state is best helped by a kapha reducing diet and many stimulating herbs. Herbs for this state can include: brahmi, shank pushpi, ginko, calamus, mint, sage, basil, sassafras, coffee, dandelion, thyme, aloe vera, garlic, golden seal, neem, guggul, and ginger root, and black pepper. These herbs are all uplifting and slightly stimulating. Use calamus powder only under the supervision of a practitioner because it is considered a poison in large doses. Exercise, especially first thing in the morning, can also help prevent the kapha predominate person from feeling lethargic.

48) Receding Gums

Cause: When dental hygiene is superb and the gums are still receding, the cause can be from the beginning stages of osteoporosis. Receding gums are sometimes due to a lack of calcium in the diet or an acidic condition of the body. The gum will shrink and recede as the tooth shrinks. Your tooth is bone matter.

Treatment: Follow the recommendations for osteoporosis in this book in section 6. Take a calcium/magnesium supplement and make sure you have 400 IU of vitamin D, and trace amounts of boron in your supplement as well, for the best absorption of the minerals. You may want to consider taking a formula that amounts to 1200 to 1500mg of calcium.

Cut back, and avoid too many acid foods such as grapefruits, lemons, cranberries, oranges, pineapple, tomatoes, pickles, sour cream, yogurt, alcohol, coffee, and kiwis. It might be wise not to drink orange juice on a daily basis, unless it is calcium fortified. Include more foods in the diet that are high in calcium and buffer acidity. Check out the section on heartburn in part 6 for ideas.

49) Ringing in the Ears

Cause: This condition is basically air and ether trapped in the ear canal. This is a wind condition, or a vata condition in Ayurvedic medicine. I have found in my practice that sometimes the ear will even itch when there is much dryness in it. As the plasma content in an individual decreases, dryness increases, sometimes giving rise to an increase in space in the channels, including the ear canals.

This change can even cause sensitivity to noise, such as the volume of a television or radio seeming "too loud" all of a sudden.

Treatment: Use heavy herbs that are moistening, heavy and considered tonics. Look for formulas with some of these herbs making up the bulk of the formula: licorice root, shatavari, ashwagandha, codonopsis root, slippery elm, vamsha rochana, bala, marshmallow, rehmannia, wild yam, Solomon's seal, ho-shou-wu, hawthorn berries and amalaki. Try 2 capsules two to three times a day until the problem is gone, or 1/2 teaspoon two to three times a day of the herbal powders in a formula. (Pittas should avoid amalaki, and hawthorn berries as they are sour). Vitamin C, A, D, and E are good oily, sour, and heavy vitamins. Also fill your ear canals with warm sesame oil everyday, then drain them. Apply several drops of oil to the inside of your nostrils as well. Include plenty of heavy, moist foods in your diet, as well as drink plenty of sweet fruit juices, and milk. Winter quashes, pumpkin, artichokes, zucchini, tomatoes/sauce, summer squashes, avocado, cucumbers, lemonade, grapefruit, kiwis, bananas, oranges, pineapple, grapes, peaches, plums, pears, melons, coconut, fresh figs, mangoes, tofu, wheat, oatmeal, rices, nuts, ice cream, yogurt, meats, and seafood are good. Avoid most herbal teas, coffee, black and green tea, as these are drying, light, and diuretic. Avoid or reduce "air" increasing foods such as: popcorn, corn chips, cornbread, rye bread, millet, buckwheat, quinoa, amaranth, broccoli, cauliflower, cabbage, Brussels sprouts, kale, collards, dandelion greens, spinach, too many salads, too many legumes/beans, peas, radishes, kohlrabi, turnips, white potatoes, burdock, and bitter and astringent herbs. Take a warm bath or swim in fresh water every day to help restore moisture to your body, soaking up to 30 minutes at a time.

50) Scanty Menstrual Blood (amenorrhea)

Cause: When a woman's menstrual period lasts only two or three days and she is not in menopause, nor does she have a cyst blocking the flow of blood, then the lack of blood usually is caused from a deficiency condition (vata imbalance). Translated, this means she is too dried up internally (yin deficient), blood deficient, lacks much nourishing substances, or her body fat has dropped too low from dieting. A mild type anemia may be associated with this or not. Lack of menstrual blood does not always mean anemia. Other symptoms of a deficient blood condition are dizziness, pale face and pale tongue, dry hair and skin. Although amenorrhea is most often a vata condition in Ayurveda, as said above, sometimes it can be due to a kapha condition such as some type of obstruction in the reproductive tract, or in pitta cases, severe liver qi stagnation that has caused the menstrual period to disappear altogether.

Treatment: Assuming the cause is due to high vata, the woman's diet needs to be very nutritive. She should emphasize plenty of vata reducing foods and herbs such as: meats, seafood, poultry, beef, pork, milk, cottage cheese, cheese, yogurt, sour cream, nuts, peanut butter, wheat, oatmeal, brown rice as starches, winter squashes, pumpkin, zucchini, summer squashes, okra, artichokes, tomato sauce, bananas, purple/green grapes, oranges, pineapple, coconut, mangoes, pears plums, peaches, kiwis, lemons, limes, molasses, brown sugar, white sugar, maple syrup, chocolate, and tofu. Avoid the sour fruits above if you are sour sensitive pitta person, dislike them, or have any heartburn, ulcers, or diarrhea.

Herbs that build blood and increase plasma/moisture are: shatavari, ho-shou-wu, cooked or raw rehmannia root, licorice, slippery elm, longan berries, lycium fruit, codonopsis, bala, amalaki, hawthorn berries, the Indian chywan-prash formula, kapikacchu, Solomon's seal, marshmallow, and wild yam. Additional herbs to add to these, to help circulate the blood are: angelica, peony root, ligusticum, and milletia root. These can be added in smaller quantities and are contraindicated in bleeding disorders or pregnancy.

51) Sinusitis

Cause: This is considered to be an infection in the sinus region/upper respiratory passages or inflammation of the sinus passages. In Ayurveda, sinusitis is a pitta disorder. Signs of an infection in the sinus cavity are green, yellow, or blood streaked phlegm and mucus.

Treatment: To stop and prevent reoccurrence of infection, consume more pitta reducing foods regularly. While the infection exists, temporarily take bitter herbs that have anti-biotic effects such as: echinacea, golden seal, neem, bhumy amalaki, gentian root, dandelion, guduchi, or bupleurum. If there is much congestion such as thick, heavy mucus being dispelled from the nose, a tea brewed from mullein leaf and peppermint can help dry up nasal secretions without aggravating inflammation. Try also taking 1/4 to 1/2 teaspoon vasaka powder (or 1 capsule) 2-3 times a day to dry up mucus. If there is dryness within the nasal passages (often in vata and pitta-vata people), a tea made of licorice, fennel, comfrey, eucalyptus, and mint can help moisten as well as open nasal passages. Use more of the fennel, comfrey and licorice in this formula, as these are the moistening herbs. Sweeten with white sugar or maple syrup. Heavy, moistening herbs for dry, inflamed nasal passages include bala, vamsha rochana, shatavari, Solomon's seal, codonopsis, marshmallow or licorice root. Vatas almost always have dry nasal passages whereas kapha type people get the severe congestion.

52) Skin Diseases (psoriasis, rosacea, eczema)

Cause: These skin disorders are caused from high pitta in the system. In Chinese medicine they are classified as a heat pattern with possible dryness or moisture. The common characteristics of these disorders are red discolorations, red patches on the face, neck, legs, torso, or arms, and sometimes peeling or flaking of the skin. Dryness coupled with red discoloration of the skin is more common in vatas, vata-pittas, and pitta-vatas. Kapha predominant people usually won't have the flaking and scaly patches, although I did see it in one of my cases due to severe heat drying out the skin. Think of psoriasis, rosacea, and eczema as a type of inflammation or infectious heat condition trapped in the skin.

Treatment: Eat more pitta reducing foods; they are cooling. Internally, take blood cleansers and herbs that drain pitta, heat, fire, infection, inflammation, and stimulate healthy liver function such as aloe vera gel, echinacea, golden seal, dandelion, yellow dock, red clover, gardenia, coptis rhizome, gentian root, neem, or bhumy amalaki. These herbs are mostly bitter, should be taken in small doses, and used temporarily until the condition clears up. Other herbs that clear heat include: lily bulb, mint, red raspberry leaf, mullein, gentian, honeysuckle flower, chrysanthemum, licorice, codonopsis, Solomon's seal, shatavari, slippery elm, and marshmallow. Pitta, and vata men and women should include some moistening herbs like licorice, shatavari or Solomon's seal, along with the bitters, to prevent themselves from becoming too dried up, physically drained, or hyperactive, as bitters can cause these effects on them. If there is dryness and flaking associated with the psoriasis, include more of those herbs in a formula, avoid soaps, and apply coconut oil topically to the skin, as well as taking baths instead of showers more frequently. For more oily psoriasis, aloe vera gel can be applied topically.

53) Sore, Achy Breasts (during or prior to the onset of your menstrual cycle)

Cause: This condition is usually due to one of two different causes: either you have liver congestion or water (swelling) of the breast tissue. If the soreness you have is due to liver congestion, you may have other symptoms such as: frequent headaches, irritability, frustration, unjustified anger, muscle and shoulder tension, genetic high cholesterol, an irregular period, and possible soreness in the abdomen over the liver area (your right hand side). Pitta, pitta-vata, and pitta-kapha women are most susceptible to this condition. If your soreness is due to swelling (some edema of the breast tissue), you will notice that your breasts increase in size right before your period. You may even have water weight gain in other areas of your body like the ankles, prior to menstruation. Kapha type women usually have this type.

Treatment for the liver congested type: Follow the recommendations under the section for an irregular menstrual cycle due to liver congestion. Including more pitta reducing foods in your diet to help the liver's energy flow more smoothly. Also try liver regulating herbs temporarily until the problem is gone. Good liver regulating herbs are bitters such as: aloe vera gel, dandelion, turmeric, guduchi, neem, golden seal, bhumy amalaki, milk thistle, red clover, echinacea, burdock root, and chrysanthemum.

For the kapha edema type: Try herbal diuretics such as uva ursi, cleavers, shilajit, parsley, dandelion, juniper berries, cornsilk, or punarnava. Take dosages depending on your height and weight. A 5 feet 10 inch, 175 lb. woman may need 2-3 capsules three a day. Whereas a 5 feet 4"

135 pound woman shouldn't use more than 2-4 capsules a day. Since all of these herbs are diuretics, use them only temporarily and cautiously since they can cause potassium depletion. Remember, you want to treat the root cause, so if you are retaining that much water, dry up your diet! Avoid moisture promoting foods: bananas, tomatoes, kiwis, lemons, limes, oranges, pineapples, coconut, melons, papaya, yogurt, sour cream, buttermilk, pickles, oatmeal, too many wheat or rice products, nuts, tofu and soy products, winter squashes, parsnips, pumpkin, artichokes, olives, zucchini, cucumbers, and too much salt. If you are kapha predominant, then a kapha reducing diet will naturally help decrease the inclination towards water retention.

54) Sore Throat

Cause: These are basically related to inflammation and infection in the body (a pitta disorder). In Chinese medicine they are viewed as part of a heat pattern. Generally, vatas will have the mildest sore throats, but also a dry throat as well; pittas will have the most severe sore throats, and kaphas will have milder sore throats with mucus, or excess phlegm in the throat.

Treatment: Emphasize more pitta reducing foods in your diet that reduce and cool inflammation, infection, and heat. Strongly avoid acidic, sour, spicy, and fermented foods such as lemons, limes, kiwis, grapefruits, orange juice, pineapple, rhubarb, sour berries, cranberries, pickles, olives, tomatoes, any vitamin C, ginger, mustard, ketchup, horseradish, curries, too much black pepper, garlic, chilies, cinnamon, coffee, alcohol, yogurt, feta cheese, buttermilk and sour cream.

Vatas, vata-pittas, pitta-vatas, and pittas can take the herbs that cool inflammation and restore moisture to a dry sore throat such as: bala, slippery elm, shatavari, Solomon's seal, or licorice root (4-6 capsules a day for a week). They can brew a tea of fennel, and coriander in equal parts to be taken three times a day with white sugar. Use 1 teaspoon of the powdered herbs per cup hot water. Stronger antibiotic, anti-flammatory, anti-heat herbs can be used temporarily such as echinacea, golden seal, or neem. Exercise caution, as these herbs are very drying. Vanilla ice cream, milk, vanilla, pudding, tofu, soda, white rice, white sugar, cucumbers, zucchini, watermelon, honeydew, Santa Claus melons, sweet red apples, pears, dates, figs, coconut milk, and purple grape juice are excellent foods for this condition as they are all cooling, sweet, and somewhat moist.

Pitta-kaphas, and kaphas can use just gentian root, bhumy amalaki, neem, echinacea, or golden seal for infection and inflammation. They can drink a tea made from peppermint, red raspberry leaf, mullein, and chrysanthemum. Sweeten the tea with honey to cut mucus. A gargle can be made out of turmeric and white sugar.

55) Sweating Excessively

Cause: Large quantities of sweat usually means one or two of these factors; you are either internally too hot/overheated and/or too internally damp. If you are too hot, you may or may not have some of these symptoms: a red colored tongue, flushed or reddened face/skin, dark yellow urine, rapid pulse, excessive thirst, huge appetite, feeling irritated, angry, frustrated, hot palms and foot soles. Dampness manifests itself in being overweight, having heavy and stiff limbs, water retention, a wet handshake, being uncomfortable in humid temperatures, feeling lethargic, and a coating on the tongue. In Chinese medicine, dampness usually moves downward first so the legs are more frequently affected in that they probably feel heavy.

Treatment: If you are truly hot, cool yourself down by increasing foods, beverages and teas that have a cooling effect on the body. See the suggestions under treatment for hot flashes. If you are damp, follow a drying diet. If you are hot and damp, emphasize foods that are both cooling and drying.

Dry foods and herbs: corn grains, rye bread, chips, buckwheat, millet, radishes, garlic, carrots, apples, pears, apricots, peaches, raisins, prunes, pomegranates, cranberries, berries, Brussels sprouts, cabbage, cauliflower, broccoli, turnips, leafy greens, coffee, grain substitute coffees, black tea, peas, legumes/all beans except soy, celery, bell peppers, corn on cob, leeks, kohlrabi, mushrooms, onions, beet greens, strawberries, burdock root, dandelion tea, lemongrass tea, mustard, chamomile tea, cinnamon teas, ginger teas, raspberry leaf tea. Natural diuretics are: uva ursi, dandelion, parsley, shilajit, cleavers, juniper berries, chickweed, punarnava.

Cool and dry foods/beverages: mint teas, chicory grain coffee substitutes, black tea, chrysanthemum flowers, lemongrass, chamomile tea, bancha twig tea, red clover, apples, pears, berries, lettuce, spinach, kale, collards, cauliflower, cabbage, broccoli, white potatoes, celery, peas, green beans, dandelion greens, raisins, prunes. Some cooling, dry herbs are: uva ursi, dandelion, cleavers, and corn-silk.

56) Tremors

Cause: Trapped air and ether (wind) in the nerve channels. When deficiency in the body is combined with air or too much lightness, a vata condition results causing tremors. However, I have also seen it in kapha-pitta people due to a Chinese condition called liver-wind. The vata deficiency type is sometimes, but not always related to Parkinson's disease. Sometimes, certain prescription drugs can also cause tremors in thin, small people, such as some anti-depressants. I had several cases in my practice where this was true. One woman who was on an anti-depressant had a tremor in her hands. The anti-depressant was over stimulating her nervous system. When she stopped the anti-depressant, the tremor went away within a month, and so did the insomnia.

Treatment: Avoid foods that are too airy. Excessive doses of B vitamins can cause or exacerbate this condition as well, and I recommend that they be avoided. Consume more vata reducing foods as these are heavier and more grounding. Decrease your consumption of leafy greens, popcorn, chips, rye breads, rice cakes, cauliflower, cabbage, broccoli, Brussels sprouts, peas, white potatoes, apples, cranberries, dried fruits, legumes/beans, cornbread, corn tortillas, corn chips, buckwheat, millet, and pears. Avoid herbal teas like chamomile and peppermint. Vata predominant individuals can also take tonic (nourishing), heavy herbs such as: licorice, rehmannia root, wild yam, codonopsis, longan berries, dates, ho-shou-wu, kapikacchu, shatavari, ashwagandha, ginseng, vitamin C, hawthorn berries, triphala, schizandra, and amalaki. These are heavy, sweet, or sour and grounding also. They help nourish the heart when there are palpitations. Use vata reducing sedatives for any insomnia: jatamansi, zizyphus, ophiopogon, and valerian if there is insomnia also. If you have menstrual irregularities, a pitta body type, or headaches, diarrhea, or heartburn, avoid the valerian, ashwagandha, hawthorn berries, amalaki, triphala, schizandra, and ginseng. Try the other herbs 1/2 tsp. 2-3 times a day in powdered form or 2 capsules 2-4 times a day. Try 1/4 - 1/2 tsp. or 1-2 capsules of the sedatives at night. Warm milk at bedtime with nutmeg and poppy seeds is a nice nerve tonic and very mild sedative.

If your condition is due to liver-wind and/or a liver-spleen condition, you may have more of these symptoms present: frequent headaches, irritability, frustration, anger, sore achy breasts right before the menstrual period if you are female, an irregular menstrual cycle, muscle or shoulder tension, bloating and gas in your abdomen, loose stools, tenderness below the rib cage especially on the right side over the liver. For the liver type of tremors, include more pitta reducing foods in your diet. Temporarily try some liver regulating herbs such as: bupleurum, turmeric, aloe vera, bhumy amalaki, lemon balm, Oregon grape root, dandelion, golden seal, or neem. You may want to look in the other areas of this book under digestive complaints such as diarrhea, etc., if poor digestion is also playing a role in your case.

57) Ulcers

Cause: These simply mean that your body is too acidic caused from either an overly acidic and spicy diet and/or your body type being predominantly pitta. Pitta dosha is clearly out of balance!

Treatment: Avoid grapefruit, lemons, limes, kiwis, papaya, rhubarb, strawberries, sour berries, cranberries, strawberries, bananas, pickles, olives, tomatoes, orange juice, pineapple, alcohol, coffee, sour cream, yogurt, feta cheese, garlic, horseradish, curry and other strong spices. The vata or pitta type person can take 1 capsule 3-4 times a day of formulas that include some of the following herbs: licorice root, marshmallow, kapikacchu, bala, slippery elm, shatavari, fennel, cumin, ho-shou-wu, dandelion, neem, golden seal, aloe vera, gentian root. The latter five herbs listed are much stronger. Kapha and kapha-pitta type people can try simply any of the following herbs: gentian root, musta, arjuna, ashoka, red clover, dandelion, neem, golden seal, or turmeric with meals, along with mint, chamomile and mullein tea. Chicory grain coffee substitutes are excellent beverages for stopping acidity in the digestive tract. White sugar, red sweet delicious apples, pears, purple grapes, dates, figs, coconut, melons, tofu, milk, vanilla ice cream, white potatoes, broccoli, cauliflower, cabbage, kale, and collards also stop acidity in the gut. Emphasize the foods here that agree with you.

58) Urinary Tract Infections

Cause: These are due to high pitta in the system. Chronic urinary infections and inflammation means your diet is too acid and you have heat in the lower burner area of the body.

Treatment: Eat more pitta (cooling/low acid) foods such as leafy greens, broccoli, cauliflower, cabbage, peas, green beans, asparagus, milk, vanilla ice cream, white rice, apples, pears, purple grapes, dates, figs, watermelon, honeydew, etc. Reduce or eliminate your intake of: grapefruit, lemons, limes, kiwis, rhubarb, strawberries, bananas, sour cream, yogurt, buttermilk, coffee, alcohol, tomatoes, oranges, pineapple, garlic, chilies, salsa, olives, and pickles. To stop infection, try strong bitters, which are natural antibiotics: gentian root, golden seal, neem, echinacea, bhumy amalaki, bupleurum, or aloe vera gel. If you are a small or thin build, such as in the case of vata or vata pitta people, use heavier herbs such as bala, shatavari, licorice root, Solomon's seal, marshmallow, or raw rehmannia root in a formula along with smaller doses of the bitters.

59) Weight Loss (unwanted)

Cause: This can be from many causes such as colitis, too much exercise, eating disorders, surgery, sickness/disease like cancer, etc. Those factors aside, it usually comes from eating too many foods and substances that contain too much "air and ether," and/or having a genetically fast metabolism. Generally, this is a vata condition, and vata people tend to have this problem. Sometimes the person is taking in a lot of substances that are naturally astringent, which not only promote the tightening of tissue, but also are diuretic and catabolic in their nature. Foods like these, literally "lighten" the body. These are cruciferous vegetables like broccoli, cauliflower, cabbage, Brussels sprouts; bitter greens, salads, beans, apples, pears, cranberries, berries; crunchy dry foods like chips of any kind; white potatoes, bell peppers, burdock root, peas, and sprouts. Sometimes too many pungent foods will do the same thing such as radishes, leeks and kohlrabi. Rye grains, buckwheat, corn, amaranth, millet and granola are light grains.

Treatment: To reverse this, omit the above foods and consume more tissue building (anabolic) foods and herbs. Foods that are naturally sweet, sour, salty, or damp promote weight gain because they contain a lot of the elements earth and water in Ayurveda. Dairy is excellent for weight gain especially ice cream, yogurt, and cottage cheese, along with wheat products, rice and oatmeal. Amino acids, protein bars, and milk or yogurt shakes with bananas, and eggs are helpful. Bananas are great for promoting weight gain, as are melons, kiwis, papaya, grapes, dates, figs, mangoes, nuts, avocado, coconut, tahini, eggs, meat, seafood, tofu/soy foods, grapefruit, oranges, pineapple, lemons, limes, sweet winter squashes, pumpkin pie, crème pies, tomatoes, artichokes, olives, pickles, zucchini, yellow summer squash, plantains, cucumbers, and sweet potatoes. Also decrease the amount of aerobic vigorous exercise you are currently doing. Substitute walking, yoga, tai-chi, or swimming, or decrease a 45 minute session of aerobics to 20 minutes no more than three times a week. Herbs that help slow metabolic activity down are the yin tonic herbs that reduce vata in the body: licorice root, marshmallow, Solomon's seal, shatavari, rehmannia, codonopsis, slippery elm.

7

Myths and Facts About Natural Eating

Seasonal Cooking and Eating

One of the best things you can do to maintain or improve your health is to eat what's in season. By doing this, you will not only save money but will adjust to the climate changes around you comfortably and help prevent seasonal flus and colds. Although cold air itself does not directly cause illness since colds and flus are caused by viruses, not cold air, it is still an external pathogen that can further weaken your system if your body type/constitution is already weakened. It can make you more susceptible to catching a virus. In Chinese medicine, developing a cold due to a change in the weather is explained as an external pernicious influence invading the body because your qi (vitality, life force, constitution) is already weakened. However, you can help minimize this chance of being affected by external influences by eating foods that are in season. For example, eating foods and substances that are cold during the winter, make it harder for the body to stay warm and dry. The result is that you get sick/discharge this energy by a cold or flu. In the summer, the opposite happens. The heat escalates and the air becomes either drier or more humid depending on where you live. Nevertheless, there is more heat. Compensating for this is very important so you do not become at risk for a heat stroke. Hence, we generally take in more cooling foods like salads, asparagus, green beans, peas, melons, juicy fruits, more liquids, ice cream, popsicles, and raw juices including lemonade and red grape juice. We can cut back on spices in our cooking to cool down as well, or emphasize cooling ones like fennel, cumin, mint, vanilla, coriander, and cilantro. The foods grown seasonally automatically help us do this.

Ever experience feeling chilled after eating ice cream or salad in the winter, or overheated in the summer after a heavy baked meal or spicy bowl of chili? Have you felt like eating artichokes in the middle of the hot humid summer? Probably not. Foods in the winter that are traditionally grown during the summer periods taste awful. It's unnatural. Many years ago, people did not have the luxury of eating out of season, because they lacked the technology we now have to store all kinds of foods, as well as ship coconuts from other parts of the world to upstate New York in the winter time. They also did not have air conditioners in the summer to compensate if they became overheated. Instead, they "lightened up" their diets in the summer and made the food more cooling by using cooling cooking methods. If you have trouble picking out the seasonal foods in your supermarket, just look for what's on sale or on display in the produce section. Some summer foods are: cherries, berries, melons, peaches, apricots, plums, mangoes, coconut, figs, green and wax beans, summer squashes, cucumbers, leafy greens, celery, avocado, rhubarb, asparagus, okra, corn on cob, zucchini, yellow summer squash, ice cream, tofu. Some winter foods are: pumpkin pie, sweet winter squashes, Brussels sprouts, cauliflower, broccoli, beets, onions, turnips, apples, pears, bananas, oranges, pineapple, grapes (the season for them is really fall), carrots, burdock root, artichokes, more salt, more meat or beans. However, not all of these foods are cooling or heating but they are seasonal and have benefits because of that.

When you vary your cooking styles you also change the energetic property of a particular food to some degree. By doing this, you help yourself stay warmer in the winter and cooler in the summer. For example, you can take a carrot which is considered a vegetable with warming properties and juice it or serve it raw in a salad, hence making it a bit cooler then had it been baked or stewed. Winter warming or "yang" cooking styles are: baking, pickling, pressure cooking, stewing, nitsuke (stir fry followed by adding some water, covering the pan and cooking the food until the water has evaporated), soup, boiling. Summer cooking styles are: frozen, juicing, raw, steaming, stir fry, and boiling. I listed boiling in both categories because boiling is neutral in its energy.

One last note about summer heat: you can stay much cooler in the summer by eating less meat. Animal meat is very heating in its energy! If you are vegetarian, in the winter season be sure to forgo the salads, ice cream, and too many fruit juices. Instead add more warming spices and salt to your dishes. Include more soups, stews and baked casseroles to maintain your balance.

Who Should Follow a Raw Foods Diet?

People always ask me what I think about raw food diets and juicing type fasts, as they are often part of a cleansing program. My answer is mixed. It depends on the nature of the individual's body type/system, their current medical condition, and the climate that they live in. People who have frail, lightweight, underweight, or thin shaped bodies, (the vata body type), should not practice a raw food diet. Raw foods, although high in live enzymes, contain a lot of air and ether, the very substances conducive to weight loss and deficiency. They also are a poor dietary choice for people suffering from anxiety as well, since anxiety in some cases is related to feeling "ungrounded" or literally a condition of excess air and ether in the nerve channels. Furthermore, raw foods are extremely hard to digest because of their cold, wet, and rock hard nature. If you are a person with weak digestion, have trouble gaining or maintaining your weight, and have poor energy, then raw foods can weaken your body. What I mean by poor digestion is: bloating, gas, constipation, or a variable appetite. (Although some cases of pitta type diarrhea do respond well to raw foods in the diet).

Furthermore, if you happen to live in a northern/cold climate, eating raw foods all the time, or too many of them, will make you feel chilled because they cool the body down internally. For some people, this type of a diet will make it impossible for them to stay warm in a northern climate, especially if they are a cold body type to begin with. People benefit most from the effects of raw foods in the summer time.

So in which cases is a raw food diet appropriate? I believe that people who are overweight respond well to an increase of raw foods in their diet, or people with a heat condition such as hot flashes and "fiery" appetites. I also think that this type of diet is good temporarily for people who are just coming off of a highly processed meat or toxic diet and lifestyle. In this particular case, they can benefit from a temporary raw food diet as part of a cleansing regime. Other people who benefit from a raw food diet are those with "excess qi" conditions (the kapha, kapha-pitta, and occasionally some pitta types). The kapha over weight types can remain the longest on such a regime since they have the most abundant tissue (muscle, fat, nerve, etc.), and stamina.

Some of the medical conditions which will be aggravated by a raw food diet are: tremors, some types of anxiety and insomnia, some types of fatigue such as fatigue due to deficiency, Parkinson's disease, hyperthyroidism, TMJ/lockjaw, and ringing in the ears. Some people with certain types of cancer may benefit from a raw foods or cleansing diet, but certainly not if the individual is already in a severely weakened, frail, or deficiency state.

How Much Water Should You Really Drink?

I felt it was necessary to address this issue since there is so much conflicting advice on this subject as well. Here is my opinion: If you practice a vegetarian diet, your requirement for drinking water will be less than that of a meat eater, because vegetables and fruits have a higher quantity of water in them to begin with. Also, if you cook up 1/3 cup oatmeal with 2/3 cup water, the oatmeal you eat for breakfast has a percentage of water in it absorbed in the cooking process. Meat, on the other hand, is much lower in its water content. Furthermore, animal meat and its high protein content act as a diuretic in the body. This is the reason why high protein diets are so attractive to many people. People lose a lot of water weight initially when they start a high protein diet, but this weight is not fat weight. On a positive note, drinking extra water temporarily fills your abdomen up, thus curbing appetite. This is beneficial to you if you are eating and snacking when you are really thirsty.

Second, if you eat a highly processed and fatty diet, drinking extra water is probably a good idea, since that type of diet is more toxic and the fat can cause platelets to clump together and become sticky. Extra water will help thin instead of thicken blood, and will also help flush nitrates and preservatives, and chemicals from your body.

Third, if you go for a run in the hot blazing sun in the middle of the day in July, drinking extra water before and after this workout will help prevent heatstroke and dehydration. It makes common sense if you physically exert yourself and spend much time in the sun and heat, to drink more water. Furthermore, people with any type of heat imbalance in the body will benefit from consuming extra water, such as those with hot flashes, certain types of skin problems like rosacea, inflammatory types of pain, feeling too hot all the time, and especially being extremely uncomfortable in hot weather. Symptoms which indicate a heat imbalance in the body also include: red face, extreme thirst and hunger, red scarlet tongue, rapid pulse, spotting between periods, and possibly dry skin.

Fourth, vata types, and people with a tendency to be dry, have a greater need for water and liquids to help build up plasma and restore moisture to all the tissues. However, drinking too much water by force feeding it can disrupt the energy of the spleen and your digestive function, not to mention create an extra burden on the kidneys. The kidneys will have to pump and filter the extra, unneeded water. Also, if you have edema (a serious medical condition in which the kidneys are not pumping out fluids in the body), drinking extra water may worsen the situation by either adding to an already damp situation or strain already weakened kidneys. Picture this: your body is retaining an abnormally large quantity of water that is jeopardizing your health, and is having trouble releasing the water due to poor kidney or spleen function, consuming too many watery-type foods, or some other reason. Will force feeding extra water help the situation? I doubt it in most cases.

All in all, I believe in drinking only when you are thirsty, not force feeding yourself eight to ten glasses of water a day, and compensating for the above mentioned circumstances. If you are a vegetarian, or eat a lot of unprocessed natural food, force drinking extra water is not always necessary.

Vegetarianism: The Controversy and the Facts

Although much scientific data has proven that vegetarians have less cancer, hypertension, and obesity than meat eaters do, I strongly believe that some people are not designed to be vegetarians. Some people simply cannot digest beans without severe bloating and gas. Furthermore, many mock soy "meats" contain fermented substances such as malt, yeast, and soy sauce, which some people cannot digest without abdominal bloating and gas. Any severe digestive disturbance does not equal health. There are others who seem to have difficulty also, because they have a physical tendency to be internally cold. Meat is very heating to the body, so in cases where it is excluded, extra salt, spices, and cooked warming foods are needed to help maintain one's balance especially during the winter months. If you happen to live in a cold northern climate, such as the northeastern portion of the United States, or have a medical condition caused from too much internal coldness, practicing a vegetarian diet might not be in your best interest. Also, as some people tend towards thinness naturally (vata predominant types), eating legumes can exacerbate this, since beans are drying, light and more conducive to weight loss. In cases of physical deficiency and weakness in the body, meat is more helpful since it is heavier and much higher in fat, calories, and protein. Deficiency diseases such as Parkinson's, osteoarthritis, anorexia, and scanty periods can be exacerbated by a vegetarian diet.

Although, do be aware that beans and whole grains, along with dairy products, eggs, soy products, and peanut butter, do contain substantial amounts of protein. In fact, the human requirement for protein is only about 40 mg a day, which can easily be met on a vegetarian diet. Most Americans consume on average about 100-120 mg a day. Furthermore, vegetarian diets tend to be higher in produce and dietary fiber, which currently are lacking in the American diet. For more information regarding the facts, contact the Earth Save Foundation in Santa Cruz California, the Physicians Committee for Responsible Medicine, PETA, or read John Robbins' book, *Diet for A New America.* My favorite vegetarian cookbooks that are very tasty yet American in the cooking style are: *The New Farm Cookbook, The Vegetarian Lunch Basket, Meatless Meals for Working People*, and *The New Laurel's Kitchen*. The recipes in these cookbooks are easy to follow and do not involve gourmet-style cooking.

In the area of nutrition, "vegans," (pure vegetarians who consume no dairy, fish, poultry, beef, eggs, etc.) need to be concerned with only one main nutrient: vitamin B-12. Vitamin B-12 is the only nutrient that doesn't exist in the plant kingdom. Some say it exists in fermented foods, but the amount is so small that I personally wouldn't count on it. However, it is found in large amounts in dairy products and eggs. Supplementing with a B-12 vitamin or a B-complex is easy to do. The body only needs about 50 mcg. per week. There are also many different types of vegetarians such as ovo lacto (those that eat eggs and dairy), or pesco vegetarians (those that eat fish as well). I have even heard of an egg o' pancake vegetarian where the person will pretty much eat a vegan diet allowing for the occasional egg in the pancake batter when dining out or in.

Vitamins and Natural Supplements:
When You Should and Should Not Take Them

As you can gather from the information in this book, I support the use of vitamins, minerals, and other natural supplements in the reversal of human disease. However, based on personal experience with my patients, my professional training and education, I also believe that each case should be weighed separately when determining if the supplements are appropriate for that individual. Vitamins and other natural supplements have different energetic properties, along with the fact that they are needed in the body in some quantity to carry out a variety of cellular functions. Despite RDI recommendations for certain nutrients, and so-called expert recommendations for higher dosages of some supplements in the prevention of cancer, longevity, and other diseases, I believe that people all have different requirements that don't necessarily fall into these categories.

Again, as stated at the beginning of this book, vitamins and other supplements have specific properties and energetics besides their obvious biological requirement and need in the human body. Many know that vitamin C increases the production of collagen in the body so it helps us maintain healthy skin and hair, connective tissue, prevents scurvy, is an anti-oxidant, and so on. However, let us not forget that vitamin C is also sour, extremely acidic, and warming in its energy. If a person has a health disorder aggravated from too much acidity such as chronic heartburn, an ulcer, or colitis, then vitamin C will only serve to aggravate these conditions. Generally speaking, vata people seem to do well with supplementing their diets with vitamin C, and papaya enzyme tablets seem to help their digestion because these substances are sour and help maintain their equilibrium. Interestingly, people who have a tendency to be more acidic than others, need less vitamin C, and seem to have a higher biological need for the minerals calcium and magnesium to buffer their acidity, and prevent diseases like osteoporosis.

All supplements affect people in different ways because we all have different body types, different digestive tracts, and different biological needs including our need for certain dosages of vitamins, minerals, and other supplements at different times in our life. Natural supplements affect the doshas in different ways. Some vitamins are considered heavier and oilier than others and thus are more beneficial for vata types, while others are considered to have more "airy" qualities. Vitamins and natural supplements with "airy or cold" qualities are going to aggravate people who have disorders caused by too much "wind" in the body especially if they take those supplements in high dosages. Megadoses of B vitamins can do this by causing tremors, and nervousness. These factors are in addition to the supplement biological requirements for human beings.

Megadosing on vitamins or natural supplements can also be quite dangerous. Too much vitamin E like 1200 IU or above, puts some people at risk for developing a cerebral hemorrhage (stroke) especially if they are also taking blood thinning drugs. Vitamin E prevents the blood from clotting and is often prescribed by doctors for heart patients or people with high cholesterol/coronary artery disease for this very reason. You need to be very cautious when combining prescription drugs with vitamins or herbs. It gets more dangerous when you do this, and is not necessarily the best idea. Everyone is different and will react differently. Also, many pitta type people get headaches from taking large doses of minerals and hence should probably avoid them.

Does Taking Vitamins Make a Difference?

More vitamins, like more herbs doesn't necessarily mean better health. During my appointments, I have met many people who were taking for years, 20 to 30 different kinds of supplements and vitamins at once, yet they still had the same health problems before they started the vitamins. I think there are several reasons for this. One main reason being the factors I just mentioned above. Another reason being that you can't pop pills of any sort and expect to get well if you don't make the changes necessary in your diet and lifestyle. It's like assuming that if you take neem or peppermint to decrease acid reflux disease, but continue to eat spicy and acidic foods. The best herbs and natural supplements in the world won't help you if the foods you are eating and the lifestyle you are living is antagonistic to your body system and medical problem. People do this and expect miracles. I strongly do not believe in the concept of the "magic pill." I have heard people claim that one pill, one vitamin, or one supplement can cure all your problems. This is simply not true. We are too different and complicated, and illness is too complicated for one pill to solve everything. If this were true, there would be many millionaires by now and we'd all be physically well.

Here's one example of this concept. One man in his early sixties called me years ago with third stage metastasized cancer (he happened to be my uncle). He asked me if just popping shark cartilage would help reverse his cancer. I told him that cancer is a very complicated disease, and that he needed to make major changes in his diet and lifestyle as well as look into emotional, environmental and spiritual issues that might be playing a role in his disease. Herbs and natural supplements may serve as an additional treatment to the other important factors I just mentioned. Putting himself on a total program would give him the best odds for eradicating his cancer, not by just popping one pill only, although there are still no guarantees. The man did not believe me, nor want to listen, and quickly changed the subject. I do not support the idea of continuing to eat lots of junk or simply the wrong stuff for one's system and then popping pills. The healing process will be slowed and/or weakened if you completely ignore your diet and other factors. This type of behavior ends up costing you more money and takes you longer to recover. But hey, that's your choice to make.

This brings another thought to mind regarding natural methods in the treatment of cancer. Although the odds of dying of cancer are considerably higher at stage three when it has metastasized, regardless of the choices you make, I have personally met and known many people who have survived third stage cancer and are alive today almost

15 years later due to the use of natural supplements, foods and herbs. Anything is possible, without being totally unrealistic in my opinion, and I like to share that philosophy with my patients. However, nothing can be completely 100% guaranteed as illness is complicated and the human body is not perfect.

The Safety of Vitamins

So what is generally safe to take beyond the RDA/RDI levels recommended? No one quite agrees 100 percent, but there are factual known levels of toxicity. Many experts, with whom I personally agree, suggest 400 IU of vitamin E, 500mg vitamin C, 10,000 IU of beta carotene (which your body will convert into vitamin A as it needs it, since A is very toxic in large amounts), 400 IU of vitamin D, B-complex at 10 or 25 mg, and 1000-1500 mg cal/mag. Please research these vitamins and dosages before applying them to your situation first! Some people, because of a particular medical condition, will need higher amounts of one vitamin or mineral over another. It all depends on the specific situation. Generally, though, water soluble vitamins like the B's and C are a little less dangerous than fat soluble ones like A, D, and E. What that means is that fat soluble vitamins tend to stay stored in the tissues and liver longer so they can build up in the body and become toxic.

Common Vitamins and Natural Supplements and Their Uses

Vitamin A/Beta Carotene are anti-oxidants as well as heating and heavy. The body converts beta carotene into vitamin A as it needs it. Vitamin A improves night vision, improves dry skin, prevents wrinkling and hair loss, boosts immunity, and loss of taste or smell is associated with a deficiency in it or with zinc in some people. Vata people tolerate it in higher amounts. It exists in large quantities in orange colored foods like cantaloupe, yams, carrots, winter squashes, and mangoes. Even some naturally colored margarines on the market contain it.

The B vitamins are cooling, and light in their properties, and therefore help reduce inflammation as well as hot flashes. Found in large quantities in whole grains, they are helpful in some cases of depression and stress, as they help the nervous system such as stimulating mental activity, preventing sluggishness, dullness. It is also argued that they help poor memory by sharpening it and may be useful in the prevention of Alzheimer's disease. However, in other cases where there is already anxiety and forgetfulness as a result of a deficient type nerve problem, they can aggravate it, causing tremors and hyperactivity. Vatas and vata-pitta people often report this to me. Pittas, pitta-kaphas, and kapha people seem to benefit most from this supplement. The B complex also helps us retrieve energy from our food by helping break down carbohydrates and helps lower homocysteine levels in the body - thought to play a role in high cholesterol. Brewer's yeast is a natural food source high in the B vitamins as well as high in iron. Lecithin is in the B family. It is basically composed of choline and insitol. Lecithin helps lower cholesterol by helping the liver emulsify it. Lecithin is also a component in brain cell and nerve sheaths. This substance might help nerve function.

Vitamin C builds collagen and connective tissue in the body. It is also an anti oxidant helping to neutralize free radicals in aging and cancer, is sour, heating, acidic and considered heavy. Since it has anti-histamine properties it is often used during colds. It also helps the body restore inner moisture, as well as softening the skin, and preventing cartilage from deteriorating. It is excellent for dry wrinkled skin and dry thinning/falling hair. It is also good for dandruff taken along with oily vitamins. In cases of deficient gastric or enzyme activity in the stomach, it helps reverse it, and can be a digestive aid. In cases of ulcers, sore throats, migraines, and colitis, it is aggravating. It definitely benefits vata people the most, and vata-pittas who seem to have a greater biological need for it. Natural food and sources are: citrus fruits, tomatoes, kiwis, red bell peppers, broccoli, amalaki, rosehips.

Vitamin D is essential for the absorption of calcium in the body. It doesn't hurt to take Vitamin D with your calcium and magnesium for the best absorption of the calcium. Make sure your vitamin D from all sources doesn't exceed 400 IU. If you habitually wear sunscreen, make sure it is in your diet, because our skin manufactures it naturally from the sun. Egg yolks, deep sea fish and fortified milk are food sources. Also remember, it is toxic in high doses, so if you take supplements, be careful!

Vitamin E is oily, heavy but helps counteract blood clotting tendencies, as well as being an anti-oxidant. Antioxidants help neutralize and prevent the accumulation of free radicals in the body, thought to play a role in cellular aging and cancer. Vitamin E also helps reduce and prevent scarring in the body. Vata types seem to do fine with this vitamin. Again, do not use it or use large amounts of it if you are on blood thinning drugs or herbs. Natural sources are high quality vegetable oils such as those expeller pressed.

Vitamin K helps stop bleeding and is abundant in leafy green vegetables as well as cauliflower.

Calcium and magnesium are used by the body, in conjunction with boron and vitamin D to help build and maintain bones and teeth. They are often taken to help slow osteoporosis. Many people I know believe that only dairy products contain large quantities of calcium. While they do contain large amounts, they are not the only sources of this mineral. Calcium is abundant in carrots, carrot juice, kale, collard greens, bok choy, lettuce, mustard greens, prunes, beans, tofu, sardines, as well as other sources. In fact, one glass of carrot juice has more calcium than one glass of cow's milk.

Chromium helps stabilize blood sugar levels in diabetics by helping regulate insulin. It is one mineral that is usually deficient in diabetics; but is also slightly stimulating to the body. It is used in some cases of depression and for weight loss. The best form to take is chromium picolinate, as it is the easiest form to absorb. Safe dosages are about 200 mcg. a day.

Selenium has been shown to help protect people from cancer and is an anti-oxidant, but in too high doses it is toxic. Moderately safe recommended dosages by most experts are 55–200 mcg. Used safely, it helps us prevent the accumulation of toxic substances in the body. Research amounts first before using it.

The food supplement chlorophyll, including alfalfa tablets, is said to aid the body in getting rid of radiation from x-rays. Whether this is true or not, I really don't know. I do know that it helps stimulate healthy liver function and is good for pitta people and cases of jaundice. It is also drying to the body and cold in its energy, as well as being light.

Bee pollen has been thought to increase energy, but because it is a pollen, it can cause acute allergic reactions and even death in some very sensitive people. If you are going to try it, make sure you do not have allergies to pollen or bees and try it in tiny doses first to test it.

Amino acids are the building blocks of protein synthesis. Because of their anabolic nature (building muscle tissue), many athletes use them especially in the sport of bodybuilding. They are better for vata people or people with deficient types of fatigue, or wasting of body or muscle tissue. In cases of cancer, I would personally avoid them since protein feeds cancer according to many alternative medicine theories.

Betaine hydrochloric acid tablets help improve digestion only in people who need it due to a lack of gastric acid and enzyme activity. In cases of colitis, heartburn, ulcers, and/or diarrhea, where there is already too much acid secretion, they exasperate the symptoms.

Acidophilus is the friendly bacteria residing in a healthy gut. Taking it can help rebuild that flora, especially after taking a round of antibiotics, which often kill it. It is also used to help treat some kinds of candida/yeast problems. However, do keep in mind that it is a sour, fermented substance that can aggravate pitta related health problems, causing indigestion, bloating, gas, and loose stools in some people.

Fatty acids such as evening primrose oil, borage oil, fish oils, and flaxseed oil help reduce vata in the body by helping to lubricate dryness in the body. They help prevent dry skin, dry hair, constipation, aid dandruff cases, as well as cracking and popping in the joints. It has been argued that fatty acids also help lower bad cholesterol (LDL), increase HDL (the good cholesterol) in the body and may decrease some types of inflammatory pain, and even some types of depression. I'm not sure I agree with this theory, as flaxseed oil is heating and in my opinion, will aggravate inflammation. They are also considered blood thinning.

Glucosamine and chrondroitin are often taken together to help prevent and repair cartilage destruction in the joints. There is both proof and debate as to how effective they really are. Cartilage destruction is often a vata disorder (deficiency), so a highly nutritive diet with much heavy, dense and moist food, along with herbs that contain these properties, will have a greater impact in the prevention of osteoarthritis. However, these supplements may be an additional measure to take.

8

21 Additional Steps You Can Take Right Now to Improve Your Health and Life

1) Avoid processed foods, foods with artificial coloring, flavoring, preservatives, and additives as often as you can.

2) When choosing starches, pick the whole grain varieties: brown rice over white, whole wheat over white breads, corn or whole wheat tortillas, real rye bread, buckwheat or whole wheat pancakes, etc.

3) If you eat beans, buy them fresh dried, instead of canned. If time and cooking them is a problem, soak them overnight in water, then pressure cook them. They are usually cooked in about fifteen minutes this way, depending on the type of legume.

4) Always buy fresh vegetables and fruits, unless the fresh fruits are too acidic for your system to handle at the moment.

5) Avoid frozen, boxed, and canned foods. Next time you want macaroni and cheese or pancakes, make them from scratch. They're almost as quick and easy. You'd be surprised. Make all your cakes, cookies and deserts from scratch too. Homemade is best. If eating out, request these items as much as you can considering what's possible.

6) Avoid aluminum in foods, baking powder, deodorants, and aluminum pots and pans. There has been controversial debates and research indicating a possible link between Alzheimer's disease and aluminum. Whether this is true or not, why take the chances?

7) Drink filtered water or spring water.

8) Decrease the amount of fatty foods you consume such as animal fats and hydrogenated oils. These are the most dangerous to the body for some people. Avocados and nuts are healthy polyunsaturated fats

that don't necessarily need to be cut back. They are considered the good fats like expeller pressed vegetable oils.

9) Consider eating organic meat and cutting back your meat consumption in general. Animals are routinely given antibiotics and other drugs to prevent disease while they are housed in factory farms. These drugs enter and stay in the tissues of the meat.

Also, toxic matter accumulates as you move up the food chain. Meats also contain nitrates, which are converted to nitrosamines in the body which are potential carcinogens. Uric acid is another toxic by-product of meat, as well as ammonia, partly responsible for causing gout.

10) Avoid the use of electric blankets, electric razors, cell phones, hair blowers, and microwave ovens. Numerous research studies have shown that these items of modern convenience contain EMFs (electromagnetic fields). There has been much discussion, controversy, and research regarding their possible unsafety when placed near the human body for prolonged periods of time. Even electric alarm clocks emit EMFs, so you do not want to place them close to your head while you sleep.

11) Get some kind of regular exercise whether it be jogging , skiing, soccer, basketball, walking, tennis or swimming, yoga, dance, tai chi. The key is to find something you like and then do it consistently.

Maybe you're the type of person who'd rather cross train for variety, challenge and to prevent boredom. Or maybe you need to sign up for a class for extra motivation. An exercise partner in the gym or walking buddy might be the incentive you need. Whatever you decide, pick something and make a commitment to it. Learn to see exercise as natural, normal, and part of your everyday routine like brushing and flossing your teeth every morning. If you are a vata type person, or have a vata imbalance, pick slower moving and non-vigorous forms of exercise like yoga, walking, tai-chi or swimming. Also limit the total amount of physical activity you engage in. Don't push yourself.

12) Have or develop skills to cope with stress. See a professional counselor for suggestions and help if you need to. In the meantime, try some of the following: exercise, talk it out with another person or persons be it friends, family, a priest, counselor, rabbi, or support group. Do something else physical: take a warm bath, go shopping, get a massage, write the situation on paper and burn it, throw darts, meditate, go for a ride in your car up into the nearby hills and let out a good yell. Get help for more ideas and training on how to relieve the stress. You need healthy outlets, everybody does! Learn to vent anger in positive constructive ways. Also, remember that stress is a state of human perception. If you work on changing your perspective about the situation, some of the stress may dissolve since your atti-

tude changed. Learn how to see the problem or demands of you differently. Maybe the problem isn't really a problem or maybe there's a good reason for the situation such as it preventing you from experiencing something worse. Perhaps something better is waiting for you down the line or a gift will come out of the event. The situation could be teaching you a new skill or showing you what you can do to improve on something.

13) Have or develop a positive attitude and an open mind. My best success cases are with patients that have both. They seem to do better than the ones who don't, and more of them actually recover! There is an old school of thought that has been said a thousand times: what you believe usually becomes true for you in most cases or ups your odds of it becoming true. Your thoughts help create and shape your future by opening doors, ideas, and motivating you to take action to get the results you want. The mind is also like a magnifying lens. If you focus on the negative aspects, those thoughts will multiply, cloud your world and you will have a bad day.

14) Never give up hope! Hope is a good thing. It keeps you persistent and persistence gets results sooner or later. Hope motivates us to take action and is a positive emotion. Action also gets results.

15) Find out what you want to do in life and then try to do it. If there are several things in life that you want

to do, pick one or two, if it's impossible for you to do them all. People that are happy tend to live longer, recover easier, and/or at least enjoy their life and what time they have on this planet. Life is short. Make what you can of it and have fun! Depending on your religious beliefs, you only go around once on this planet earth in your current form–so have fun now!!!

16) Be kind and considerate to people. There is enough violence, jealousy, and hatred in this world. Plus, being a decent human being to others makes you feel good. Hey, why not feel good? That's why you're reading this book, to feel good, right? When you make other people feel good it has a domino effect and they make others around them feel good. The whole world can feel good!

17) Turn life over. Do what you can to remedy the situation then let it go. Turn it over to the universe, your God, whomever or whatever to worry for you. Then let it go. It's not worth as much as you think. In 20 – 30 years from now it may or may not really matter. Then again it might. So ask yourself, will this matter in 20 years from now? If not, let it go.

18) In the midst of chaos, keep it simple. Do one thing at a time, then simplify your life. It helps make sense out of a chaotic situation and helps keep your sanity. The more you have and the more you have going on, the more you have to worry about in your

life. You are likely to reach mental gridlock. One exception to this suggestion: if chaos makes you feel good, then keep it.

19) Allow yourself to be a dreamer. Some people actually make their dreams a reality. Dreams allow us to indulge the mind in a blissful state, provided they don't cause us to focus on what we don't have and make us feel self pity. Dream like there's no tomorrow. Dream happy dreams. Visualize wonderful and good things. It keeps the spirit alive inside you! Dreaming is a powerful motivator and motivation causes you to take action to get the results you want.

20) Always be grateful for what you already have. This attitude allows you to feel somewhat at peace with your current surroundings. It also makes life more tolerable and enjoyable. It helps you keep the focus on what's positive in your life.

21) Have a lot of faith or belief in what you are doing. The body follows the mind. Your mind helps create physiological changes. It also helps either stimulate or squelch ideas propelling you to take action. Keep believing, keep acting and never give up!

9

Emotional Health

Living Mentally "Free"

Since there is a strong relationship between disease and our emotional state, I strongly believe that happiness is one of our necessities. Living life the way we want to, is one major factor in creating this, and what I refer to as living mentally "free." The other is having fun. How many of us adults still look forward to waking up in the morning, and can honestly say we love what we are doing? For most of us, our lives and behaviors are molded into what "society" and others think is best, or right for us. We have also played a personal role in the making of our own lifestyle and beliefs. However, most of us don't even know what we may be missing out on, or what we could be experiencing, if our perspectives, thought patterns, and actions were to change.

For starters, we need to do two things. First, we need to be fully human. Second, we need to reprogram our thinking. What do I mean by being fully human? To be human means to fully experience the world in the physical sense, by being creative, playing, using all of the five senses, and using our mental faculties. We all are born into this world with a sense of curiosity, happiness and creativity. Creativity is part of the learning process of children. We explore our worlds physically and mentally by splashing in muddy rain puddles, play with our bare feet in the sandbox, lie on our backs watching the clouds float in the sky, build tree forts, etc. To watch a flock of geese cross the sky, spot a full moon, or even watch seeds sprout in a jar, is fascinating! Roller coasters are breathtaking, and sledding after the first snow fall is exhilarating. We look forward to many things such as the shear joy of swimming in a pond or the ocean. We "play" while still discovering our world. We read books, learn new skills, build things, make things, mimic adults, defy adults, take risks. Life is an adventure. We look forward each day to what we might discover or experience. We laugh when we want to and cry when we need to. We fully use our senses: we "touch" our world and "see" new things and "hear" new sounds. We "taste" new foods. We learn what rain "smells" like. And when we are small, the only thing that matters to us, or is most important, is having our basic human needs met: love, food, oxygen, clothing, warmth, and shelter. We have few worries beyond that. Life is simple. That is being human.

Then one day the whole picture begins to change, and life becomes this complex web of politics, economics, social status, competition, etc., far beyond the basic needs for survival. It starts in school, where we are taught to color inside the lines and not to shout and get excited "out loud." Boys are taught not to cry and girls aren't suppose to love weight lifting, auto mechanics, or carpentry. We grow up learning that it is "un-cool" to do certain things. We are too old to trick or treat. We quit collecting icicles and don't have time to ride our bikes. Our bare feet never touch the earth again. Even though our interest in things change as we age, many of us forgo the willingness and openness to continue to "explore" our world altogether. Some of us won't give ourselves permission to just "be" or be "us." We learn new codes of proper behavior. We learn to perceive our world based on other people's reactions to ourselves and our situations. As a result, some of us end up choosing careers or jobs that are expected of us, instead of following our wildest dreams. As we spend more time working, our behavior may be molded even more to company politics, and all this begins to take something away from us. Our creativity and sense of exploration of the self and world begins to dwindle. Our true identity gets buried, our sense of spirit dies, or we cease to have fun. There are things that we have convinced ourselves of, that prohibit us from living our life the way we want to and are meant to.

We are no longer mentally free when we believe and act this way. Our lives have become this doldrum. We become complainers, negative in our thinking, unexcited about anything, tired, bored, and unhappy. Why shouldn't we, life after all is about routine and responsibility. What have we to look forward to? We have to go to work and pay the bills. There are all these crises and constraints in our lives now. Life is serious and complicated. It's about status, income, what groups or cliques we belong to, or what we do or do not get invited to. Life is about who said what or did that, or what image you didn't live up to.

While we do have responsibilities that we didn't as children, it doesn't mean we can't have fun or make the time for fun. It doesn't mean we can't experience the world a little differently, and begin to do the things we truly want to. Having fun and continuing to explore your world doesn't have to be difficult or tedious, expensive or even time consuming either. It can be as simply as jogging your normal route in reverse direction to see the landscape or houses from a different angle. It can mean driving home a different way from work so that your scenery changes, or saying yes to something that you've said no to before, or no to something you've always said yes to. It can mean learning a new skill, taking a new class at night, or a weekend seminar. As said before, it may even mean slowing down and doing nothing for a day. When was the last time we took a deep, long "pause." Let the dishes go for one night, or the yard work go for one weekend and take a time out. Put on some soothing music, or go out dancing, or hiking on the weekend. Maybe take a visit to a park, or place you've never been to.

When was the last time on a Saturday or on your way home from work that you stopped off somewhere and did something that deviated from your routine? When was the last time that you played in your yard (if you have one), instead of working in it, or took a relaxing bath instead of a shower? Life is short. We are on a time limit. Take and make the time to enjoy life and do some things you want to! If you've always wanted a motorcycle and can afford it, get a license and go out and buy one. What are you waiting for?

As I said earlier, one of the reasons that keep some of us from living and doing what we want to are the belief systems we created. Author Anthony Robbins, in his book *Unlimited Power*, has said that we become comfortable in our set behaviors, because feeling and perceiving this way is familiar to us. We have thought this way our whole lives. He has also said that, unfortunately, we are either taught self help tools that enforce positive aspects of our life and thinking, or negative points. And we have habitually trained our mind to focus on either the positive aspects of our day, or the negative downside. It has been said before by numerous different people that the mind amplifies whatever you focus on. Furthermore, our beliefs and dreams help create and shape our world. Anthony Robbins states that they do this by either motivating us to take action towards reaching our goals, or not. He goes on to suggest that when our mind is open in a favorable positive direction, we create a medium in which to grow ideas to the solutions to situations. The current beliefs you hold may be what others have, but are they right for you? Are they working for you? Are they helping you to get the results you want in life? What would happen if you didn't follow them? Maybe you are afraid of success. It might mean that your life could change a bit. That can be scary, but it could mean the results you end up with are more rewarding and better than you ever imagined. It certainly does take more courage to stand up for what we truly believe in deep down inside of us, take action, and hence create change. But when we do, we set the ball rolling and are set free. It's like cleaning out a closet and getting rid of all the junk or skeletons, and then spreading your wings and flying and seeing new things. The destination could be fantastic.

Years ago I decided I didn't want a conventional job working for someone else, doing something I didn't love regardless of the salary. I decided if I was miserable, it wouldn't be worth it. No job would be worth the pay if I hated it. I wanted a profession where I didn't have to compromise my own values and beliefs. So I decided to go back to school for a third time, study alternative medicine, then go out and practice my passion, and become self-employed. So what if I got a late start in life because I changed fields a couple of times. I didn't care, and I don't care if anybody does care.

The point is, we all have to live with the decisions we make, and beliefs we hold. Nobody will live it for us, despite the fact that they may want to tell us how to go about it. I also strongly believe that if we want something bad enough, put all our efforts into it, and if it is meant to be, the universe has a way of making it happen. It just may not be on our time table, or quite when we want it. On the other hand, if what we are doing is not bringing in the outcome we desire, maybe we are barking up the wrong tree, or we need to change the type of action we are taking, as Tony has often suggested.

Never ever give up, and never succumb to negative thoughts when trying to achieve something. I finally gave myself permission to follow my passion, which I had always thought of as just a hobby or an impossible reality. I decided what my priorities were, then chose to build my life around them. I asked myself on many occasions, what steps can I take to get closer to my dream? Then I took them, one by one.

There are no rules in society besides breaking the law. The only rules we have are the ones we created inside our heads from other people's influences, people's reactions to us, our own unique take on that information, and our past experiences. The rules you define and create your life around, can be either be constraining or freeing. If you like the ones you've adopted, keep them. If not, give them up one by one and replace them with different ones, as said by author Tony Robbins in: *Unlimited Power*. We have two options: redefine our current life the way we want to some degree, or change our attitude towards it.

Start by surrounding yourself with positive people or people that make you feel good about yourself! This helps build up self esteem when it is weakened. There is another old saying that if you play a game of tennis with someone who plays worse than you do, your tennis skills decline. If you hang around depressed people, you become depressed too. So the second suggestion is: hang out with positive people and life gets more fun. Suggestion number 3: then live your life the best way you possibly can, doing what you want as you are able to. Start by taking small steps towards your goal. Throw or give away any material things or belief systems you don't like. Then create your own. Jump up and down and shout "yeah" when you get excited. That is being free! And by feeling mentally free, we are able to release more easily: resentment, anger and negative emotions that stress our minds. Living in the positive and having fun helps relax us, relaxes our muscles, and keeps our immune systems strong. Having a stronger immune system helps prevent disease. When our mind and spirits soar, we recover from illness quicker and better. And if for some reason we don't recover from illness, our quality of life was better, and life was worth living! Set yourself free! You do not have to make major life changes. Even one small thing makes a difference, and it gets you a little closer to being where you want to be, and being who you want to be!

Ways to End the Downward Spiral of Depression

Depression is worth mentioning here because I believe it can get in the way of letting you feel and be mentally free. We all know depression has an environmental and mental component, as well as a physical cause. I will address primarily the environmental and mental one below. (For the physical cause, see "depression" in part 6 of this book.)

Depression is complicated because there are so many reasons and circumstances for its cause. Everything from dissastifying relationships, jobs and home environments, to having a physical/chemical imbalance or hurtful childhood issues can contribute to it. Depression is also a funny thing. It can keep you locked in the unbearable situation that has caused you to be depressed or unsatisfied with your life in the first place. It's a viscious cycle. It prevents us from realizing our dreams and moving our life in a forward direction. I call depression a "suck zone," like in the movie *Twister*: It literally sucks you in and keeps you swallowed up in what feels like a black hole. It's a cycle of insanity where the individual keeps doing the same things over and over again, gets the same results, but then repeats those same actions. The person gets stuck on an emotion that reinforces certain patterned thoughts that feed the emotion and vice versa. Feeling "depressed" then, leaves the person feeling so exhausted that they do not have the energy to make the necessary changes to get out of the trench they are in. I have found that there are several ways to help break out of this, depending on the complexity of the issue.

1) Get involved in some temporary professional counseling to help you see through the situation to the solution, and help you change behaviors and thoughts that keep you stuck in depression. Counseling can also help make sanity out of the insanity you seem to be experiencing. (I have always thought of counseling, not for the sick, but for the healthy sane individuals that happen to be sensitive people reacting in a normal way to an insane environment. On the other hand, people do practice insane behaviors and counseling is excellent for learning new behaviors that help stop disorders such as compulsive obsession, alcoholism, drugs, eating disorders, anxiety, etc.). Professional counseling can also help you deal with childhood or past issues that may be affecting how you see and live in the world as an adult. Our thought patterns and processes form when we are children, and are literally a

sum total of all our life experiences up until this very moment. Professional counseling help can be a major step, as you remove skeletons from your closet, rebuild your self esteem, and/or create new behavior and thought patterns on which to live a healthy and satisfying life.

2) Do something different to snap yourself out of these train of thoughts. After all, depression is really a pattern way of thinking. To break out of it, you need to cut the tape, so to speak, that reverberates in your head. This can be done in many different ways. Anthony Robbins, in his book: *Unlimited Power*, suggests when thinking or feeling a certain way, pick an event or memory from the past or a fantasy from the future that makes you feel great, and blow up this image or feeling in your mind and body so that your focus shifts. You are basically replacing negative emotions and thoughts with positive ones. Anthony Robbins also suggests creating a scene in your mind that is pleasing. For example, I have fond memories of being on the beaches in Connecticut and on Long Island where I spent part of my childhood. I remember sitting on the deck of our boat with the wind blowing across my face, the hot sun beating down on my scalp, and the incredible view of the ocean stretching on forever. I also remember a time when I won a medal from running a track meet in high school and placing second.

You can also cut the tape by getting up and moving to another room while in this thinking mode, or getting in your car and going someplace you haven't been. A physical change of scenery is good. Pick a different route to drive home from work if it's possible. Perhaps you have an activity that makes you feel good that you can participate in when your thinking heads towards depression. Mine is shopping. Do not listen to any pieces of music or watch any movies that feed or trigger this downward spiral. Change the radio station. Put in a different CD. Pick one that makes you feel great, not one that feeds this already somber mood. If you are tired, put on some stimulating music; if anxious, put on something calming, and so on. You can literally use your environment to psychologically tricking your mind into thinking that it is happy and excited. Do something completely different! If you have a picture on your living room wall that triggers emotions or memories that don't make you feel well, get rid of it! Get a picture that reinforces feeling good!

3) Despite the difficulty, try to see your situation from another perspective, if changing the situation is impossible. This helps keep your attitude in the positive, instead of the negative. Every situation has another perspective. Human emotions are based in part on the perspectives we hold of the situation, along with the mental images we keep in relationship to the situation. If we work on changing the image and perspective, it gets harder to feel "down," especially if we replace the negative image with a positive one.

4) Rely on outside help to find out all your options, get the answers you need, and the solutions to the problems you have. For example, I knew a woman who was going through a divorce who realized her part time job was not enough to support herself on. Yet she didn't have all the formal education to make a career change. She was unhappy in her job anyhow, and realized what she really

wanted was a career in health administration, not just nursing. So she went to a local college to find out what programs they offered and what kind of financial aid packages she could receive. What had originally been a hellish of a situation, as she put it, going through a painful divorce, ended up turning into a refreshing change that gave her a new start on life.

Another woman I know felt financially poor being self-employed with no retirement, personal savings, or company 401K plan to fall back on. However, she was able to save 200 dollars a month, by cutting back on several expenses, and deciding not to buy a new car. Instead she chose to drive an older car with a good record, and cheaper car insurance. She used that extra money to invest in some good mutual funds with interest rate returns of about 23% (at a time when the market was good). She did her research on mutual funds with the help of several friends she had in the business sector. She also received a small inheritance of 5,000 and within several years, had turned a little bit of money into a lot of money. She kept reinvesting the interest she made as well as adding to the original existing funds.

5) Work on building up and maintaining your self esteem. Low self esteem often plays a role in depression, and depression can contribute to low self esteem, depending on the circumstances you are involved in. For example, we can justify negative circumstances and reinforce them by telling ourselves lies such as: "I always have bad luck, it'll never happen," "I'm not smart enough anyway," "I'm not good enough, so of course I can't do it." You can learn to counteract your negative thoughts with positive

ones, as suggested by Louise Hay in *You Can Heal Your Life.* Professional counseling can also help with this, as well as help you discover where these self-doubts and criticisms are coming from.

Also, try surrounding yourself with positive people who treat you decently. You deserve to be treated decently. We are all gifts on this planet. Select good friends. Many people with low self esteem seem to attract people in their lives that don't treat them very well. They are used as doormats. As self esteem increases, you realize one day that you deserve better, and start asking why you should be treated so terribly. The energy around you changes and better people start coming into your life. Also learn to say "no" when you want and need to, and "yes" when you want. As your own personal boundaries and self esteem improve, so will the ability to say "yes" and "no." Learn to be able to confront people, if that is an issue with you. Healthy self esteem allows you to be able to stand up for yourself, love yourself, and be able to feel good about yourself on a regular basis.

Louise Hay, as well as several others, have published several excellent self help books that can be a big help to you. Several favorite books of mine are: *You Can Heal Your Life*, by Louise Hay, *and How to Be Your Own Best Friend*, by Mildred Newman and Bernard Berkowitz. Talk show host, Sally Jesse Raphael once said that she had been fired numerous times before becoming successful on TV. Each time she was fired, she would tell herself that the employers just didn't appreciate the type of talent she had to offer. She told herself, she deserved much better, and the "fit" was just wrong.

6) Be persistent, yet different. If what you are doing doesn't work, try again, but this time try a different avenue. Tony Robbins has said in "*Unlimited Power*," that the main difference between successful people and ordinary people, is that successful people keep trying different things until they get the results they want. They never give up, but keep changing the type of actions they make until one type yields results. If one shoe doesn't fit, try another.

7) Get regular exercise if you can. Exercise releases endorphins, natural opiates, as well as helping to "lift" the emotions. When people look good and feel physically strong, they tend to be less depressed.

8) Do not lump every event that seems negative together in the same pot. Try to see the whole picture. For example, if your relationship is on the rocks, you just got a speeding ticket, and your kid at school got in trouble recently, try to focus on the positive aspects in your life that are going on at the same time as these misfortunes. Make a gratitude list. Try not to come to the conclusion that your life is going to pots because of these three incidents. What about all the good stuff that is happening recently in your life? The gratitude list will help you see it.

9) Pay attention to the other emotions feeding into your depression. Many people I know aren't just depressed, but have much built up anger, resentment, loneliness, frustration, or self pity tied in with their anger. If this is the case, also work on outlets for these other emotions. There are many ways to deal with anger such as: confronting the person(s) or situation you are angry about; doing physical activities to release the energy from the

pent up anger such as boxing, hitting a pillow or tree with a stick, running into the woods or meadow and letting out a good yell, etc; learning to see the person you are angry about as a "sick" individual, which makes it harder to for you to feel animosity towards him/her; asking yourself if you set yourself up because of having certain expectations that didn't come through, or were you selfish in your motives. Often, we get angry because people and life situations don't turn out as we expected them to, as if we were some kind of God, having the power to control all of life's forces and people. We can control so much up to a point, and then it becomes necessary to "let go" or "go with the flow," like doing the dead man's float in a river. On the other hand, if a situation didn't turn out like you wanted to, maybe you should try a different kind of action until you get the results you want, or change your goals or perspective of the situation.

Picking up the phone and calling a friend or relative just to chat can combat loneliness. You can also make a conscious effort to get out more often in public, by getting involved in clubs, church groups, group activities, joining a gym, attending a lecture at a nearby college, or simply going to a mall or supermarket where lots of people congregate. Any of these experiences can be social as you meet new people. People are also funny in their behavior. Sometimes you have to make an extra effort to get together with them by calling the first shots such as inviting them over for dinner. Volunteering for a good cause, organization, or charity is another way to meet and be around people.

Unfortunately self pity gets us nowhere and in the least direction. It keeps us stuck and almost paralyzed, preventing us from taking any further action. It also prevents us from making the appropriate decisions necessary that may help us get out of the situation. However, we are human and could all use a good hug every now and then. Sometimes I believe the world could be much more loving. My advice is to get your hugs, cries and kisses, then get busy to take your mind off of the situation. Do an activity that is fun, upbeat and positive. Go see an inspirational film! Go shopping, go for a hike, visit a museum, do anything and something that is fun to you. There are many steps one can take to start alleviating depression. This book lists only a few to get the ball rolling. Despite the fact that depression can be a nasty cycle, it can also be a learning tool, by pointing out just where our life needs to change!

Last Words

If there is anything at all that you have learned from this book, I hope it is the fact that the "miracle cure/pill" does not exist. Furthermore, what's indeed "healthy" is a relative term. There is no such thing as tofu, miso, or yogurt being healthy for everyone, nor should ginseng, mega doses of vitamin C, echinacea, and St. John's Wort be recommended for every single person. The key to perfect health and living a satisfied life is different for everyone. There is no one magic solution. One cannot give "generalized" treatment recommendations across the board for everyone, nor suggest how everyone should spend their lives. We are all special, biologically and psychologically unique. Our medical conditions have different causes, many different variables involved, and we are complex beings. We must match recovery plans with these factors.

Without doing so, the results we desire, are not likely to happen.

However, I strongly believe that recovery is possible for more people than they realize, and alternative medicine can treat more disorders than what most people think. I am always blown away in my practice by the types and amount of medical problems that go into complete remission using natural medicine. Being alive is truly a gift, and being a human being who is alive and well, is even a greater gift. We have so many things which we have created in this world, in which to experience. Time is short in this form. Enjoy the ride before it ends! I hope to have deepened your insight on healing the human body and mind, and have made your journey a little less difficult!

May health become your greatest wealth. Best regards!

Pat O'Brien

Suggested Reading

Bensky, Ted and Andrew Gamble. *Chinese Herbal Medicine: Materia Medica*. Washington: Eastland Press, 1986; 1993.

Fan, Warner J-W., M.D. *A Manual of Chinese Herbal Medicine, Principles and Practice for Easy Reference*. Boston: Shambhala Publications, Inc., 1988.

Frawley, Dr. David and Dr. Vasant Lad. *The Yoga of Herbs*. Wisconsin: Lotus Press, 1986.

Griffith, H. Winter, M.D. *The Complete Guide to Prescription and Nonprescription Drugs*. New York: The Berkeley Publishing Group, 1983; 2001.

Hay, Louise. *You Can Heal Your Life*. Santa Monica, CA: Hay House, Inc., 1984.

Kushi, Michio. *Your Face Never Lies*. Wayne, NJ: Avery Publishing Group, Inc., 1983.

Lieberman, Shari, Ph.D., and Nancy Brunig. *The Real Vitamin and Mineral Book*. New York: Avery Publishing Group, 1997.

Newman, Mildred and Bernard Berkowitz with Jean Owen. *How To Be Your Own Best Friend.* Wayne, NJ: Avery Publishing Group, Inc., 1971.

Robbins, John. *Diet For A New America.* Walpole, NH: Stillpoint Publishing, 1987.

Tierra, Michael, C.A., N.D. *Planetary Herbology.* Twin Lakes, Wisconsin: Lotus Press, 1988.

Tirtha, Swami Sada Shiva. *The Ayurveda Encyclopedia: Natural Secrets to Healing, Prevention, and Longevity.* Bayville, NY: The Ayurveda Holistic Center Press, 1988.

Index

B

C

D

E

H

I

M

N

O

P

Q

R

S

T

W

Y

Z